Anesthesiology

SPECIALTY BOARD REVIEW

Anesthesiology

9th Edition

610
Questions & Answers

Thomas J. DeKornfeld, MD
Theodore J. Sanford, Jr., MD
Department of Anesthesiology
The University of Michigan Medical School
Ann Arbor, Michigan

MEPC
Medical Examination
Publishing Company

APPLETON & LANGE
Norwalk, Connecticut

Notice: The authors and the publisher of this volume have taken care to make certain that the doses of drugs and schedules of treatment are correct and compatible with the standards generally accepted at the time of publication. Nevertheless, as new information becomes available, changes in treatment and in the use of drugs become necessary. The reader is advised to carefully consult the instruction and information material included in the package insert of each drug or therapeutic agent before administration. This advice is especially important when using new or infrequently used drugs. The publisher disclaims any liability, loss, injury, or damage incurred as a consequence, directly or indirectly, or the use and application of any of the contents of the volume.

Copyright © 1995 by Appleton & Lange
A Simon & Schuster Company
Copyright © 1991 by Appleton & Lange

All rights reserved. This book, or any parts thereof, may not be used or reproduced in any manner without written permission. For information, address Appleton & Lange, 25 Van Zant Street, East Norwalk, Connecticut 06855.

95 96 97 98 / 10 9 8 7 6 5 4 3 2 1

Prentice Hall International (UK) Limited, *London*
Prentice Hall of Australia Pty. Limited, *Sydney*
Prentice Hall Canada, Inc., *Toronto*
Prentice Hall Hispanoamericana, S. A., *Mexico*
Prentice Hall of India Private Limited, *New Delhi*
Prentice Hall of Japan, Inc., *Tokyo*
Simon & Schuster Asia Pte., Ltd., *Singapore*
Editora Prentice Hall do Brasil Ltda., *Rio de Janeiro*
Prentice Hall, *Englewood Cliffs, New Jersey*

ISBN 0-8385-0256-3

ISBN: 0-8385-0256-3
ISSN: 1078-6805

Acquisitions Editor: J. Alex Schwartz
Production Service: Rainbow Graphics

PRINTED IN THE UNITED STATES OF AMERICA

Contributors

Crider, Bruce A., MD, Assistant Professor—Anesthesia for Vascular Surgery, The University of Michigan Medical School, Ann Arbor, Michigan

DeKornfeld, Thomas J., MD, Professor Emeritus, Editor—Anatomy, Physiology, Pharmacology, Medicolegal and Ethical Issues, Anesthesia for Thoracic Surgery, Anesthesia for Plastic and Reconstructive Surgery, The University of Michigan Medical School, Ann Arbor, Michigan

Dowling, Catherine A., MD, Instructor—Anesthesia for Urological Surgery, The University of Michigan Medical School, Ann Arbor, Michigan

Learned, David W., MD, Assistant Professor—Anesthesia for General Surgery, The University of Michigan Medical School, Ann Arbor, Michigan

Levy, Loren, MD, Assistant Professor—Anesthesia for Gynecological Surgery, The University of Michigan Medical School, Ann Arbor, Michigan

Mathai, Marykutty, MD, Assistant Professor—Anesthesia for Ear, Nose, and Throat Surgery, The University of Michigan Medical School, Ann Arbor, Michigan

McLaren, Ian Douglas, MB, FFARCS, Assistant Professor—Anesthesia for Orthopedic Surgery, The University of Michigan Medical School, Ann Arbor, Michigan

Mullin, Vildan, MD, Associate Professor, Anesthesia for Neurologic Surgery, Pain Management, The University of Michigan Medical School, Ann Arbor, Michigan

Murad, Sharlet, MD, Assistant Professor—Anesthesia for Ophthalmologic Surgery, The University of Michigan Medical School, Ann Arbor, Michigan

Murray, Jeffrey R., MD, Lecturer—Anesthesia for Cardiac Surgery, The University of Michigan Medical School, Ann Arbor, Michigan

Naughton, Norah N., MD, Assistant Professor—Anesthesia for Obstetrics, The University of Michigan Medical School, Ann Arbor, Michigan

Sanford, Theodore J., Jr., MD, Professor and Associate Chair—Editor, Biochemistry, The University of Michigan Medical School, Ann Arbor, Michigan

Szocik, James F., MD, Assistant Professor—Physics, Equipment and Monitoring, Anesthesia for Transplant Surgery, The University of Michigan Medical School, Ann Arbor, Michigan

Tremper, Kevin K., PhD, MD, Professor and Chair—Physics, Equipment and Monitoring, The University of Michigan Medical School, Ann Arbor, Michigan

Woodcock, Brian J., MB, ChB, FRCA Assistant Professor—ICU, The University of Michigan Medical School, Ann Arbor, Michigan

Contents

Preface vii

- 1. Anatomy 1
     Answers and Discussion 6
- 2. Physiology 13
     Answers and Discussion 18
- 3. Pharmacology 28
     Answers and Discussion 33
- 4. Biochemistry 42
     Answers and Discussion 53
- 5. Physics, Equipment, and Monitoring 63
     Answers and Discussion 72
- 6. Anesthesia for General Surgery 82
     Answers and Discussion 89
- 7. Anesthesia for Orthopedic Surgery 98
     Answers and Discussion 106
- 8. Anesthesia for Gynecological Surgery 114
     Answers and Discussion 122
- 9. Anesthesia for Ear, Nose, and Throat and Oral Surgery 130
     Answers and Discussion 137
- 10. Anesthesia for Plastic and Reconstructive Surgery 144
      Answers and Discussion 147

- 11. Anesthesia for Thoracic Surgery 151
  Answers and Discussion 156

  12. Anesthesia for Cardiac Surgery 164
  Answers and Discussion 172

  13. Anesthesia for Vascular Surgery 186
  Answers and Discussion 193

  14. Anesthesia for Neurologic Surgery 204
  Answers and Discussion 212

- 15. Pain Management 221
  Answers and Discussion 231

  16. Anesthesia for Urologic Surgery 241
  Answers and Discussion 247

  17. Anesthesia for Ophthalmologic Surgery 255
  Answers and Discussion 262

  18. Anesthesia for Transplant Surgery 270
  Answers and Discussion 277

  19. Anesthesia for Obstetrics 283
  Answers and Discussion 291

  20. Anesthesia for Pediatric Surgery 306
  Answers and Discussion 315

  21. Intensive Care Unit 323
  Answers and Discussion 331

  22. Medicolegal and Ethical Issues 340
  Answers and Discussion 344

References 349
Glossary of Abbreviations 353

Preface

The very good reception of the previous edition of this book has encouraged both the publisher and the members of the Department of Anesthesiology at the University of Michigan to prepare a new edition. Accordingly, the Ninth Edition is hereby presented to the residents, fellows, and practitioners in anesthesiology.

This edition takes a somewhat different approach. After abridged sections on anatomy, physiology, biochemistry, and pharmacology, the book is divided into chapters on the basis of the various surgical disciplines we serve. Thus, we have sections on anesthesia for general surgery, for orthopedics, for gynecology, and so on. This will make it easier for the readers to concentrate on specific areas of anesthesiology and will allow them to study the various subsets in anesthesiology in detail and depth.

Since techniques and problems tend to overlap and since the same surgical procedure may be performed by surgeons belonging to different disciplines, it became impossible to eliminate all apparent duplications. Several surgical procedures form the basis of some questions in both vascular and neuroanesthesia. They are presented, however, from the perspective of the individual specialties, and thus the answer and the discussion may vary somewhat from one specialty to the next. A review of the specific references should clarify whatever doubt may arise.

As far as the discussions are concerned, the individual contributors were given wide discretion in formulating both the content and the length of their answers. Although they were asked to rely heavily on the references they cite for each question, they were also encouraged to feel free to make comments based on their wide experience in their field of particular competence. We sincerely trust that you will find this book interesting, useful, and, occasionally, entertaining.

Thomas J. DeKornfeld and Theodore J. Sanford, Jr.
Ann Arbor, Michigan
June, 1994

1
Anatomy

DIRECTIONS (Questions 1–10): Each of the questions or incomplete statements below is followed by five suggested answers or completions. Select the **one** that is best in each case.

---

1. The cerebral arterial circle (of Willis) is composed of
   A. anterior and posterior cerebral arteries
   B. anterior and posterior meningeal arteries
   C. internal and external carotid arteries
   D. vertebral and basilar arteries
   E. posterior communicating and middle cerebral arteries

2. The spinal dura in the adult ends at
   A. S_{2-3}
   B. $T_{12}-L_1$
   C. first coccygeal segment
   D. S_{3-4}
   E. L_4

3. The nail bed of the fourth finger (ring finger) receives its sensory innervation from the
   A. median and radial nerves
   B. radial and ulnar nerves
   C. median and ulnar nerves
   D. median nerve only
   E. ulnar nerve only

4. In the adult the spinal cord ends at the
   A. fourth lumbar vertebra
   B. L_{3-4} interspace
   C. twelfth thoracic vertebra
   D. second lumbar vertebra
   E. T_{12}–L_1 interspace

5. Which of the following intrinsic muscles of the larynx is innervated by the external laryngeal nerve?
   A. cricothyroid
   B. posterior cricoarytenoid
   C. lateral cricoarytenoid
   D. arytenoid
   E. thyroarytenoid

6. The vocal cords are shortened and relaxed by which of the following intrinsic muscles of the larynx?
   A. lateral cricoarytenoid
   B. posterior cricoarytenoid
   C. anterior cricoarytenoid
   D. cricothyroid
   E. thyroarytenoid

7. The sensory innervation of the larynx is provided almost exclusively by the
   A. interarytenoid nerve
   B. superior laryngeal nerve
   C. glossopharyngeal nerve
   D. internal laryngeal nerve
   E. lateral laryngeal nerve

8. The tongue is drawn upward and backward by the
   A. styloglossus muscle
   B. genioglossus muscle
   C. chondroglossus muscle
   D. thyroglossus muscle
   E. digastric muscle

9. Which of the following is NOT a branch of the sciatic nerve?
   A. tibial nerve
   B. common peroneal nerve
   C. medial sural cutaneous nerve
   D. saphenous nerve
   E. medial plantar nerve

10. Which of the following cranial nerves is purely efferent?
    A. olfactory
    B. abducent
    C. hypoglossal
    D. trigeminal
    E. trochlear

DIRECTIONS (Questions 11–20): For each of the questions or incomplete answers below, **one** or **more** of the answers or completions are correct. Select
   A. if only 1, 2, and 3 are correct
   B. if only 1 and 3 are correct
   C. if only 2 and 4 are correct
   D. if only 4 is correct
   E. if all are correct

---

11. The blood supply to the esophagus is provided by the
    1. thyroid artery
    2. inferior phrenic artery
    3. left gastric artery
    4. bronchial artery

12. The relationships of the second part of the axillary artery are
    1. anterior to the posterior cord of the brachial plexus
    2. medial to the medial cord of the brachial plexus
    3. medial to the lateral cord of the brachial plexus
    4. central to the axillary sheath

13. The left bronchial artery
    1. is usually a single vessel
    2. arises from the thoracic aorta
    3. arises from the third posterior intercostal artery
    4. sends branches to the esophagus

14. The right coronary artery
    1. arises behind the anterior aortic sinus
    2. provides blood to the S-A node
    3. sends a posterior interventricular branch to both ventricles
    4. sends a circumflex branch along the right coronary sulcus

15. The sympathetic nervous system
    1. forms the celiac ganglion
    2. has its ganglia close to the target organs
    3. is known as the thoracolumbar system
    4. has myelinated postganglionic fibers

16. Which of the following is (are) lined with pseudostratified, ciliated, columnar epithelium?
    1. proximal esophagus
    2. nasal cavity
    3. urinary bladder
    4. lobular bronchiole

17. Which of the following are components of the lateral wall of the nose?
    1. uncinate process
    2. hiatus semilunaris
    3. bulla ethmoidalis
    4. ostium maxillare

18. The branches of the internal iliac artery include the
   1. inferior epigastric artery
   2. deep iliac circumflex artery
   3. ovarian artery
   4. uterine artery

19. Which of the following is (are) branch(es) of the external carotid artery?
   1. lingual artery
   2. superficial temporal artery
   3. maxillary artery
   4. ophthalmic artery

20. The sinuses of the dura mater include
   1. superior sagittal sinus
   2. straight sinus
   3. transverse sinus
   4. occipital sinus

Anatomy

Answers and Discussion

The authors have made every effort to thoroughly verify the answers to the questions that appear on the preceding pages. As in any text, however, some inaccuracies and ambiguities may occur. If in doubt, please consult the indicated reference. When no page number(s) are cited, the reference is to a journal article or to a refresher course lecture that should be read in its entirety.

The Editors

1. **(A)** The internal carotid and vertebral arteries provide the entire cerebral blood supply. They anastomose in the circle of Willis at the base of the cerebrum, caudad from the hypothalamus. The anterior cerebral branches of the internal carotid are connected to each other by the anterior communicating artery. Posteriorly they are connected to the basilar arteries via the posterior cerebral arteries and the posterior communicating artery. This system serves to equalize the blood flow to the different parts of the brain, even though the pressure in the internal carotid and the vertebral arteries may vary. The middle and posterior cerebral arteries originate from the circle. They are functionally end-arteries, and hence obstruction will lead almost inevitably to ischemia and very likely to infarction of the brain areas they supply. **(Ref. 18,** pp. 748–749)

2. **(C)** The dural sac proper extends from the foramen magnum to the second sacral vertebra. It does, however, continue all the way

to the second coccygeal segment as an investment of the external filum terminale of the spinal cord. Thus, the end of the dura is at the same level in both infants and adults. It is only the spinal cord that changes its relative length from infancy to adulthood. The spinal dura is a continuation of the inner (meningeal) layer of the cranial dura. The outer (periosteal) layer is attached at the foramen magnum and thus delimits the cranial extent of the epidural space. (**Ref. 18,** pp. 1088–1089)

3. **(C)** This is the only finger on which the nail bed receives its sensory innervation from two of the terminal branches of the brachial plexus. The same area of the fifth (little) finger is innervated by the ulnar nerve only, whereas the thumb, index, and middle fingers receive their sensory innervation at the nail beds from the median nerve alone. The radial nerve supplies sensory nerve endings to the dorsum of the hand on the medial side, proximal to the distal phalanx. (**Ref. 18,** p. 1132)

4. **(D)** The end of the spinal cord, the tip of the conus medullaris, is found in the adult at the cranial border of the second lumbar vertebra. At birth, the spinal cord extends to the third lumbar vertebra. This fact is of considerable importance when a lumbar puncture is contemplated in an infant or very young child. In the adult the spinal cord gives the appearance of having been "pulled" craniad, and the nerves emerging from the lower spinal segments extend caudally within the dural sac to form the cauda equina (horse's tail). (**Ref. 18,** p. 922)

5. **(A)** This is the only intrinsic muscle of the larynx that is innervated by the external laryngeal branch of the vagus (X). All the other intrinsic muscles of the larynx receive their innervation from the recurrent laryngeal nerve. All the nerves to the larynx are branches of the vagus. They include the internal and external branches of the superior laryngeal nerve and the recurrent laryngeal nerve. (**Ref. 18,** p. 1258)

6. **(E)** This is a complex muscle that has two parts with slightly different attachments and directions of pull. The main part causes the arytenoid muscles to move forward and thus shorten and relax the vocal cords. The lateral portion of this muscle rotates the arytenoid cartilage toward the midline and thus narrows the glottic

chink. The second, smaller, part of this muscle acts on the vocal ligaments. It is referred to as the "aryvocalis muscle" and is considered by some to be responsible for the control of pitch. It accomplishes this by regulating the length of the vibrating parts of the cords. (**Ref. 18,** pp. 126–127)

7. **(D)** Practically the entire sensory innervation of the larynx is derived from the internal laryngeal nerve. This is a branch of the superior laryngeal nerve. The other branch of the same nerve is the external laryngeal nerve The superior laryngeal nerve itself is a branch of the vagus. Some infraglottic sensory fibers come from the inferior laryngeal nerve which is the terminal branch of the recurrent laryngeal nerve. This one is also a branch of the vagus. (**Ref. 18,** p. 1258)

8. **(A)** The tongue is an extremely complex, muscular organ that can move in a number of directions. Protrusion of the tongue is accomplished by the genioglossus muscle. The anterior fibers of the same muscle retract the tongue into the oral cavity. Both fiber groups acting together can make the superior surface of the tongue into a groove that facilitates the passage of liquids during the sucking maneuver. The hypoglossi pull the tongue downward and depress the lateral margins. There are also intrinsic muscles of the tongue. These are the superior and inferior longitudinal muscles, the transverse muscle, and the vertical muscle. Their role is primarily to change the shape of the tongue. This function is important in making the tongue sufficiently mobile and able to alter its shape, so that it can actively participate in the formation and enunciation of sound. All the muscles of the tongue are innervated by the hypoglossal nerve. (**Ref. 18,** p. 1322)

9. **(D)** The saphenous nerve is a branch of the femoral nerve and hence comes from $L_{2,3,4}$. The sciatic nerve and its two major branches, the tibial nerve and the common peroneal nerve, originate from $L_{3,4}$ and $S_{1,2,3}$. These roots form the sacral plexus, and the sciatic nerve is by far its major component. Actually, the sciatic nerve consists of two clearly identifiable components, the tibial and the common peroneal nerves that run together in a common sheath and together constitute the sciatic nerve. The common peroneal originates from $L_{4,5}$, $S_{1,2}$, while the tibial nerve origi-

nates from $L_{4,5}$ and $S_{1,2,3}$. The medial sural nerve and the medial plantar nerve are branches of the tibial nerve. The tibial and common peroneal nerves supply the skin of the foot and most of the lower leg. They provide motor fibers to all the muscles of the lower leg and foot and to the posterior muscles of the thigh. The sciatic nerve is by far the largest nerve in the body. (**Ref. 18,** pp. 145–148)

10. **(C)** Two cranial nerves are exclusively efferent: the hypoglossal (XII) and the accessory (XI). Three are purely afferent: the olfactory (I), the optic (II), and the vestibulo-cochlear (VIII). All the others have both afferent and efferent components. The oculomotor (III), the trochlear (IV), and the abducent (VI) have motor and proprioceptive fibers. All the others (V, VII, IX, X) have motor, sensory, and visceral fibers. (**Ref. 18,** pp. 1094 et seq.)

11. **(E)** The esophagus is very richly supplied with blood from branches of the thyrocervical trunk, the thoracic aorta, and the abdominal aorta. The venous return is via the inferior thyroid, azygos, hemiazygos, and gastric veins. There is thus a rich anastomotic network between the portal venous system and the systemic venous system that explains the vulnerability of the esophagus in cases of portal hypertension. Esophageal venous varicosities and the ensuing hemorrhage are the hallmark of hepatic cirrhosis. (**Ref. 18,** p. 1333)

12. **(B)** The second part of the axillary artery is no longer in the axillary sheath. It is surrounded laterally, medially, and dorsally by the respective cords of the brachial plexus that separate it from the axillary vein and adjacent muscles. The axillary artery is the direct continuation of the subclavian artery. It is divided into three parts that are located respectively proximal to, below, and distal to the pectoralis minor muscle. Understanding the relationship of the brachial plexus to the three parts of the axillary artery is important for the proper performance of the axillary block. (**Ref. 18,** pp. 756–757)

13. **(C)** There are usually two left bronchial arteries. They originate from the thoracic aorta at the level of T_5 and just below the left main stem bronchus. They, together with the single left pulmonary artery, supply the bronchial tree, the connective tissues of

the lung, and the bronchial lymph nodes. They send branches to the esophagus and to the pericardium. The bronchial arteries form a capillary network which, at the level of the alveoli, anastomoses with the capillary network of the pulmonary circulation. (**Ref. 18,** pp. 764, 1285)

14. (**A**)　The right coronary artery is dominant in 85% of the population. In 5% the right and left are approximately equal. The left coronary artery is dominant in only about 10% of the cases. The right coronary artery supplies the S-A node in 70% of the cases and the A-V node in 92%. There are numerous variations in the configuration and dominance of the two vessels. The anterior interventricular and circumflex arteries are branches of the left coronary artery. The marginal and posterior interventricular branches originate from the right coronary artery. The two vessels anastomose with each other near the apex of the heart. (**Ref. 18,** pp. 727–731)

15. (**B**)　This division of the autonomic nervous system is characterized by the outflow from the thoracolumbar portion of the spinal cord. Its preganglionic fibers are short and myelinated, the ganglia are central, and the long, postganglionic fibers are usually nonmyelinated. The sympathetic fibers frequently run in parallel with the parasympathetic fibers and are generally antagonistic to them. The organs reached by the sympathetic fibers include the eye, the heart, smooth muscles, the GI and GU tracts and the glands, both endocrine and exocrine all over the body. (**Ref. 18,** pp. 1156 et seq.)

16. (**C**)　Only the respiratory tract has this type of epithelium. It plays a critical role in the transport of the mucous blanket and in removing small particulate matter from the airways. The nasal cavity is still part of the conducting system of the upper airways. When the motion of the cilia is decreased or abolished, respiratory complications inevitably ensue.

　　The esophagus is lined with stratified squamous epithelium, and the urinary bladder is lined by transitional epithelium. This latter type of epithelium allows for rapid and considerable changes in the volume of the hollow viscus. (**Ref. 18,** pp. 1332, 1266, 1418)

17. **(E)** The medial wall of the nose is a simple bony and cartilaginous septum, but the lateral wall is an extremely complicated structure containing all the above components. It also serves as the base for the three (occasionally four) conchae and for the entry of the lacrimal duct. The ostia to the maxillary, ethmoid, sphenoid, and frontal sinuses open into the lateral wall of the nose. The nasal cavity is roughly divided into a superior or olfactory region and an inferior or respiratory region. The olfactory nerve endings are located on the superior (supreme) concha and on the adjacent superior portion of the nasal septum.

    The nasal cavity is separated from the orbit and from the cranial cavity by very thin bony plates. Trauma may easily produce a communication between these three areas. (**Ref. 18,** pp. 1172–1173)

18. **(D)** The ovarian artery originates directly from the abdominal aorta. The inferior epigastric and deep iliac circumflex arteries are branches of the external iliac artery. The branches of the internal iliac artery are the umbilical, inferior vesical, middle rectal, uterine, vaginal, internal pudendal, iliolumbar, lateral sacral, superior gluteal, and inferior gluteal arteries.

    There is good anastomosis between the ovarian and uterine arteries and a number of other vessels from the aorta, from the deep femoral artery and the branches of the iliac arteries. Ligation of the internal iliac artery will not deprive the pelvic organs of blood supply. (**Ref. 18,** pp. 777 et seq.)

19. **(A)** The ophthalmic artery is a branch of the internal carotid. The other three are branches of the external carotid, which also gives rise to the superior thyroid, ascending pharyngeal, facial, occipital, and posterior auricular arteries. The internal carotid artery provides the blood supply of much of the brain, the orbital structures, and part of the forehead and the nose. All other parts of the face are supplied by the external carotid artery. At the bifurcation of the common carotid artery, we find the carotid body and the carotid sinus. These two structures, one extrinsic and one intrinsic to the vessel, are important in the detection of hypoxia and in the regulation of systemic blood pressure. (**Ref. 18,** pp. 736 et seq.)

20. (E) All these and the inferior sagittal sinus, the sigmoid sinus, the petrosquamous sinuses, and the confluence of sinuses belong to the posterosuperior group of sinuses. The anteroinferior group consists of the cavernous sinuses, the sphenoparietal sinuses, the intercavernous sinus, the superior and inferior petrosal sinuses, and the basilar plexus. These components of the dura are venous channels that carry venous blood from the brain and from the cranial bones to the internal jugular vein. They have no valves, but their endothelium is identical with that of the veins into which they empty. The superior sagittal sinus communicates with irregular venous spaces, the so-called lateral venous lacunae. These latter contain numerous arachnoid granules (Pacchionian bodies), which communicate with the subarachnoid space and allow cerebrospinal fluid to enter the venous system directly. (**Ref. 18,** pp. 799–804)

2
Physiology

DIRECTIONS (Questions 21–30): Each of the questions or incomplete statements below is followed by five suggested answers or completions. Select the **one** that is best in each case.

---

21. Respiratory control can be exerted by the carotid bodies. They are activated by
    A. decreased hydrogen ion concentration
    B. increased $PaCO_2$
    C. increased MAP
    D. increased PaO_2
    E. decreased MAP

22. Peripheral chemoreceptors are not significantly activated until the PaO_2 has fallen below
    A. 80 mm Hg
    B. 70 mm Hg
    C. 60 mm Hg
    D. 50 mm Hg
    E. 40 mm Hg

13

23. Systemic arterial blood pressure is increased by
    A. increased intracranial pressure
    B. decreased intracranial pressure
    C. increased arterial oxygen tension
    D. decreased arterial carbon dioxide tension
    E. increased cerebral blood flow

24. In Stage I of slow-wave sleep, the EEG pattern changes from
    A. delta to alpha waves
    B. theta to delta waves
    C. alpha to beta waves
    D. alpha to delta and theta waves
    E. rapid alpha to slow alpha waves

25. Lower extremity somatosensory-evoked potential monitoring is most useful in
    A. temporal craniotomy
    B. cochlear implant procedure
    C. diagnosing early retinopathy
    D. hearing tests in small children
    E. scoliosis surgery

26. Somatosensory-evoked potential testing is a useful diagnostic test in all of the following EXCEPT
    A. localizing spinal lesions
    B. Friedreich's ataxia
    C. multiple sclerosis
    D. acute craniocerebral trauma
    E. brain death

27. The energy used to transport Ca^{++} out of the cells is directly linked to
    A. the hydrolysis of creatine phosphate
    B. the hydolysis of ATP
    C. the influx of chloride ions
    D. the electron transport chain
    E. osmosis

28. Antidiuretic hormone production is decreased by
    A. increased baroreceptor activity
    B. decreased baroreceptor activity
    C. increased chemoreceptor activity
    D. decreased chemoreceptor activity
    E. decreased extracellular volume

29. Which of the following hormones act on the cells of the renal tubules to increase sodium reabsorption?
    A. renin
    B. cortisol
    C. ADH
    D. aldosterone
    E. angiotensin II

30. Relaxation of a contracted muscle fiber is initiated by
    A. energized myosin binding to actin
    B. removal of Ca^{++} from troponin
    C. ATP binding to tropomyosin
    D. Ca^{++} binding to calmodulin
    E. increased Na, K-ATPase activity

DIRECTIONS (Questions 31–44): For each of the questions or incomplete statements below, **one** or **more** of the answers or completions given is correct. Select
   A. if only 1, 2, and 3 are correct
   B. if only 1 and 3 are correct
   C. if only 2 and 4 are correct
   D. if only 4 is correct
   E. if all are correct

---

31. Tetanic contractions are characteristic of certain muscles. Cardiac muscle cannot generate tetanic contractions because
    1. the cytosolic Ca^{++} is too low
    2. the cytosolic Ca^{++} is too high
    3. it has a syncytial organization
    4. it has a long refractory period

32. The lung is primarily an organ of respiration. It also has several non-respiratory functions. These include
    1. releasing histamine
    2. inactivating paracrine agents
    3. converting angiotensin I to angiotensin II
    4. inactivating epinephrine

33. The body's response to high-altitude hypoxia includes
    1. hyperventilation induced by increased peripheral chemoreceptor activity
    2. increased erythropoietin secretion
    3. increased 2,3-DPG
    4. decreased 2,3-DPG

34. The eicosanoids include
    1. the leukotrienes
    2. baradykinin
    3. the cyclic endoperoxides
    4. adenyl cyclase

35. The physiologic changes caused by the aging process include
    1. decrease in limb muscle mass
    2. loss of memory
    3. difficulty in learning new tasks
    4. decreased cardiac output

36. In performing pulmonary function tests
    1. reduced FEV_1 indicates restrictive pulmonary disease
    2. in emphysema FEV_1 is likely to be less than 80%
    3. the FEV_1/FVC ratio is increased in restrictive lung disease
    4. all standard PFTs require active patient participation

37. Carbon dioxide is transported in the blood
    1. dissolved in the plasma
    2. as bicarbonate
    3. as carbaminohemoglobin
    4. dissolved in erythrocytes

38. The gastrointestinal hormones include
    1. secretin
    2. cholecystokinin

3. gastrin
   4. aminopeptidase

39. Insulin production is stimulated by
    1. increase of blood glucose concentration
    2. increased amino acid concentration in the plasma
    3. parasympathetic stimulation of the pancreas
    4. gastric inhibitory peptide (GIP)

40. The effects of glucagon include
    1. decreased gluconeogenesis
    2. decreased ketone production
    3. increased amino acid take-up
    4. increased glycogen breakdown

41. Plasma cholesterol
    1. is required for the synthesis of plasma membranes
    2. varies inversely with cholesterol synthesis in the liver
    3. is carried by low-density lipoproteins to the cells
    4. is carried by high-density lipoproteins to the liver

42. The major effects of growth hormone are
    1. stimulation of protein synthesis
    2. inducement of bone cell differentiation
    3. anti-insulin activity
    4. depression of gluconeogenesis

43. The functions of the thyroid hormone include
    1. maturation of the nervous system of the fetus
    2. increased oxygen consumption and heat production
    3. facilitation of the functions of the sympathetic nervous system
    4. depression of the production of growth hormone

44. The rate of heat production is controlled by a change in
    1. metabolic rate
    2. shivering thermogenesis
    3. sweating
    4. nonshivering thermogenesis

Physiology

Answers and Discussion

The authors have made every effort to throughly verify the answers to the questions that appear on the preceding pages. As in any text, however, some inaccuracies and ambiguities may occur. If in doubt, please consult the indicated reference. When no page number(s) are cited, the reference is to a journal article or to a refresher course lecture that should be read in its entirety.

The Editors

21. (B) The carotid and aortic bodies are located respectively at the bifurcation of the common carotid arteries and on the arch of the aorta. They are known as the peripheral chemoreceptors and are in intimate contact with these vessels. The carotid bodies are the more important group. They consist of epithelium-like cells and nerve endings. The afferent fibers go to the brain stem where their stimulus affects the inspiratory neurons of the medulla.

The peripheral chemoreceptors are in the proximity of the baroreceptors but are quite distinct from them. The chemoreceptors are not activated by changes in arterial blood pressure. They are activated by low arterial PO_2, increased hydrogen ion concentration and, slightly, by increased $PaCO_2$. The increased $PaCO_2$ acts as a stimulant primarily through the secondary changes in pH. (**Ref. 43,** pp. 500–501)

22. (C) It can be shown experimentally that if the $PaCO_2$ is controlled by absorption of the expired CO_2, and the inspired O_2 concentration is progressively lowered, the peripheral chemoreceptors will be activated as soon as the PaO_2 drops below 60 mm Hg. The respiratory rate will increase significantly in an attempt to increase the PaO_2. The reason the chemoreceptors become activated only when the PaO_2 drops below 60 mm Hg becomes obvious from inspection of the oxygen dissociation curve. It can be seen that the sharp decline of the curve begins at about 60 mm Hg and that beyond that point even slight changes in PO_2 cause a very significant change in hemoglobin saturation.

The chemoreceptors are activated by low PaO_2 and not by low total oxygen content. Hence, patients with even severe anemia, who have an essentially normal oxygen tension, will not activate the peripheral chemoreceptor. (**Ref. 43,** pp. 501–502)

23. (A) A number of cardiovascular reflexes affect systemic blood pressure. An increase in blood pressure may be produced by all of the following: decreased PaO_2, increased $PaCO_2$, increased intracranial pressure, decreased cerebral blood flow, and integumental pain.

Increased intracranial pressure reflexly raises the MAP to compensate for decreased cerebral blood flow. The increased MAP is an attempt to maintain "normal" cerebral perfusion. (**Ref. 43,** p. 459)

24. (D) Beta waves (faster than 13 Hz) are characteristic of alert wakefulness. During relaxed wakefulness, the beta rhythm changes to alpha (8 to 13 Hz) rhythm, which is maintained at an increasingly slower rate until the onset of sleep. During the first of the four slow-wave sleep stages, the waves change from alpha to theta (4 to 8 Hz) and delta (< 4 Hz). There may still be some alpha activity. By the time stages 3 and 4 set in, the delta waves predominate.

This phase is followed by "paradoxical" or "rapid eye movement (REM)" sleep during which the EEG again resumes alpha wave-like activity. This is a very similar pattern to the one seen during alert wakefulness. The REM sleep episodes alternate with the slow wave sleep periods. Each cycle lasts 90 to 100 minutes. (**Ref. 43,** pp. 272–273)

25. **(E)** The use of somatosensory-evoked potential (SEP) monitoring has become a standard technique during most scoliosis repair procedures. It is particularly useful during the Harrington rod placement. The best nerve to stimulate is the tibial at the ankle, because this area is usually accessible during the surgical procedure. Bilateral stimulation is rarely indicated. The electrodes should be placed on the side where damage during the corrective procedure is more likely. The SEP may be recorded from the scalp, neck, or epidural space, above and below the surgical site.

If the amplitude decreases by 50% or more, the surgeon must be alerted since the implications of this change may be serious. If the responses disappear entirely, the surgical procedure must be stopped immediately and corrective measures must be taken, provided, of course, that a control measurement confirms the absence of the response. (**Ref. 31,** pp. 151–152)

26. **(E)** Sensory-evoked potentials (SEP) are not useful in establishing brain death, since one of the definitions of brain death includes the absence of all brain stem function. SEP monitors only cortical functions. Although loss of all cortical function, combined with evidence of loss of medulla oblongata functions, are strong presumptive evidence of brain death, it leaves the door open for some, or even reasonably complete brain stem activity. To detect brain stem death, brain stem auditory-evoked potentials must be used. The advantage of the latter technique is that in contrast to cortical potentials it is not sensitive to drugs, alcohol, hypothermia, or metabolic or hypoxic effects. (**Ref. 31,** pp. 48, 173)

27. **(B)** Four primary, active transport enzymes derive their energy directly from the hydrolysis of ATP. These are the Na-, K-ATPase which transports sodium and potassium; the Ca-ATPase, which transports calcium; the H-ATPase, which transports hydrogen ions; and H-,K-ATPase, which carries both hydrogen ions and potassium. Na-,K-ATPase is located in the plasma membrane. The other three are located in the plasma membranes and in several organelle membranes, including the membrane of the mitochondria. It is the active transport of calcium by the Ca-ATPase, which is responsible for the low calcium concentration in the cytosol and the high calcium concentration in the extracellular fluid. The ratio is approximately 1:1000 (10^{-7} mol/L and 10^{-3} mol/L respectively).

All these transports are proteins (enzymes) that catalyze the breakdown of ATP. In the process the transporter becomes phosphorylated and this changes the translocation process. (**Ref. 43,** pp. 127–128)

28. (A) Antidiuretic hormone (ADH), produced by a group of hypothalamic cells, is the primary agent in controlling total body water. Total body water is a function of renal reabsorption of water, rather than of glomerular filtration, and it is the ADH that regulates the tubular reabsorption of water.

   Whenever the extracellular volume rises, baroreceptor activity increases, and this results in the decrease of ADH production. This in turn decreases the permeability of the collecting duct, increases urine production, and, ultimately, decreases extracellular volume.

   An additional important process, tending to work in the same direction, is the decrease in aldosterone production as a consequence of the increased extracellular water. This process is mediated by the renin-angiotensin system. A parallel process in controlling body water is mediated by the hypothalamic osmoreceptors that respond to a decrease in body fluid osmolality. Increased firing by the osmoreceptors also increases ADH production. (**Ref. 43,** pp. 540–541)

29. (D) Aldosterone is the major factor in determining the rate of sodium reabsorption in the renal tubules. Aldosterone, secreted by the adrenal cortex, regulates the absorption of sodium only in the cortical collecting ducts. Aldosterone controls only 2% of the total sodium reabsorbed, whereas 98% of sodium is absorbed by the more proximal parts of the renal tubules that are not under aldosterone control. When there is no circulating aldosterone, none of this 2% fraction is absorbed, while conversely, if there is an excess of circulating aldosterone, none of this sodium fraction is lost. Aldosterone acts by promoting the production of several proteins in its target cells, including Na,K-ATPase, that leads to active transport of sodium across the tubular epithelium. Aldosterone secretion is stimulated by angiotensin II, which is derived from angiotensin I by the action of renin. (**Ref. 43,** p. 536)

30. **(B)** There are 14 steps in the sequence of events between the arrival of the motor neuron action potential and skeletal muscle fiber contraction. These are, in an abridged form: (1) Arrival of the axon potential at the axon terminal; (2) release of ACh from the terminal at the neuromuscular junction; (3) ACh diffuses to the motor endplate; (4) ACh binds to receptor sites Na^+ and K^+ channels; (5) Na^+ and K^+ cross the fiber, generating an endplate potential; (6) adjacent plasma membrane is depolarized, generating an action potential that travels on the surface of the fiber along the transverse tubules; (7) action potential releases Ca^{++} from the lateral sacs of the sarcoplasmic reticulum; (8) Ca^{++} binds to troponin, causing tropomyosin to move away from the blocking position and uncovering cross-bridge binding sites on actin; (9) energized myosin cross-bridges on thick filaments bind to actin; (10) cross-bridge binding triggers release of stored energy, producing an angular movement at each cross-bridge; (11) ATP binds to myosin, breaking the linkage between actin and myosin, allowing cross-bridges to dissociate from actin; (12) ATP bound to myosin is split, transferring energy to myosin cross-bridge; (13) cross-bridges repeat steps 9 to 12. This will continue as long as Ca^{++} remains bound to troponin; (14) cytosolic Ca^{++} is decreased as Ca^{++} is actively transported into sarcoplasmic reticulum by Ca-ATPase.

The removal of Ca^{++} from troponin restores the blocking action of tropomyosin, the cross-bridge cycle comes to a halt, and the muscle fiber relaxes. (**Ref. 43**, p. 319)

31. **(D)** In skeletal muscle the refractory period is short (1 to 2 ms), whereas the contraction elicited by a single action potential lasts 20 to 100 ms. Thus, a second contraction can be triggered before the first one is completely over. This results in a summation of contractions that ultimately produces a tetanic contraction. In cardiac muscle the refractory period lasts almost as long as the original contraction (approximately 250 ms). Thus, stimulation during this refractory period produces no re-excitation of the fiber. By the end of the refractory period, when excitation is again possible, the muscle has relaxed. For this reason no summation of contractions is possible, and the cardiac muscle will not produce a tetanic contraction (which is just as well). This, incidentally, is one of the important physiologic differences between cardiac and skeletal muscle. (**Ref. 43**, p. 416)

32. **(E)** The lung has significant, nonrespiratory functions. It deactivates circulating substances (e.g., epinephrine) and also produces substances, such as surfactant and the angiotensin-converting enzyme which catalyzes the conversion of angiotensin I to angiotensin II.

One of the most important nonrespiratory functions of the lungs is their key role in filtering out noncellular particulate matter from the circulation. Blood clots, fat, amniotic fluid debris, gas bubbles, and other particulate matter reach the lung via the pulmonary arteries and are then trapped, depending on size, either in a branch of the pulmonary artery or in the pulmonary capillary network. Depending on the extent of the vascular obstruction, pulmonary embolism may be negligible and undetectable, or massive and rapidly fatal.

In minor and clinically insignificant embolization, the same particulate matter, on reaching the arterial side of the circulation, could and would lead to disastrous central nervous system (CNS), cardiac, or systemic infarction. (**Ref. 43,** p. 509)

33. **(A)** An increase in 2,3-DPG shifts the hemoglobin dissociation curve to the right, thus facilitating oxygen unloading in the tissues. This is a mixed blessing, since a shift to the right makes the loading with oxygen in the lungs more difficult. In fact, the increase in DPG may be counterproductive and maladaptive.

Other adaptive mechanisms include the increases in capillary density, mitochondria, and muscle myoglobin. All of these increase oxygen transfer. Increased peripheral chemoreceptor activity also stimulates increased Na^+ and water loss. This will reduce plasma volume and result in increasing the blood concentration of erythrocytes and hemoglobin.

The diuretic effects of the adaptive mechanism are too slow to prevent the acute pulmonary edema that is occasionally a life-threatening component of mountain sickness. The mechanism of this pulmonary edema has not yet been established. (**Ref. 43,** pp. 508–509)

34. **(B)** The eicosanoids are important local chemical messengers. These substances are all derived from the polyunsaturated fatty acid, arachidonic acid, which is one of the plasma membrane phospholipids. The eicosanoids also include the prostaglandins and the thromboxanes.

The eicosanoids play a large number of very important roles, and their activity is critical to the proper functioning of the body. They are significant components in blood coagulation, in regulating smooth muscle contraction, in many areas of the reproductive system, in neurotransmitter release and activity control, in hormone secretion, and in the body's response to injury and infection.

The production of eicosanoids is severely curtailed and even abolished by aspirin and by the non-aspirin, non-steroidal antiinflammatory agents. (**Ref. 43,** pp. 160–161)

35. (A) The aging process causes a number of changes, such as the loss of limb muscle mass (30% to 40%), loss of memory, difficulty in learning new tasks, and loss of brain mass. There is also a general loss of cells. Recent studies indicate that aging, per se, does not decrease cardiac output and does not decrease intelligence. If there is a change in intelligence and/or cardiac output, this is likely due to co-existing disease or a change in life-style.

    The etiology of the aging process is unclear and much debated. One hypothesis blames aging on an accumulated injury to the macromolecules in the cells. Another hypothesis alleges that aging is programmed in our genes by heredity and that the lapse of a period of time activates these genes and initiates the aging process. (**Ref. 43,** pp. 154–155)

36. (C) Pulmonary function studies, if performed correctly by a trained and experienced person, have considerable diagnostic and prognostic significance. Vital capacity (VC) is decreased in restrictive pulmonary disease and is normal or increased in obstructive disease. The PFTs are useful in following the patient's pulmonary status and in identifying improvements or deterioration in pulmonary functions. The prognostic usefulness of PFTs is largely limited to trying to predict whether a patient would tolerate major resectional pulmonary surgery.

    The problem with all standard pulmonary function tests is that they are largely dependent on the patient's willingness and ability to cooperate, as well as on the technician's experience and ability to obtain maximum and consistent effort on the part of the patient. There is considerable inter-rater variability, and unless you know how and by whom the PFT results were obtained, their clinical usefulness is limited. (**Ref. 43,** p. 486)

37. (E) Carbon dioxide is much more soluble than oxygen and hence the blood can carry considerably more dissolved CO_2 than O_2. Carbon dioxide is carried as dissolved CO_2 in both plasma and erythrocytes (10%). Thirty percent is carried as a carbamino compound with hemoglobin ($HbCO_2$). This reaction is made more readily available by the fact that reduced hemoglobin (deoxyhemoglobin) has a higher affinity for carbon dioxide than does oxyhemoglobin. The rest of the carbon dioxide (60%) is carried as bicarbonate. This reaction is catalyzed by carbonic anhydrase. The end products of the reaction are bicarbonate and hydrogen ions. The bicarbonate ion is actively transported out of the erythrocyte and is replaced, ion for ion, by chloride. This is known as the chloride shift. (**Ref. 43,** pp. 498–499)

38. (A) There are only four substances that meet all the criteria for being a true GI hormone. They are all peptides. Gastrin is produced by the endocrine cells in the antrum of the stomach. Amino acids and peptides in the stomach and vagal stimulation trigger its release. Cholecystokinin is secreted by the small intestine. It potentiates the secretion from the pancreas, contracts the gallbladder, and relaxes the sphincter of Oddi. Secretin is produced in the small intestine under the stimulation of acid in this area. It inhibits gastric emptying and stimulates bicarbonate secretion by the pancreatic and hepatic ducts. It has no effect on the gallbladder or on the lower GI tract. The glucose-dependent insulinotropic peptide (GIP) is also produced in the small intestine under the stimulation of glucose and fat. It stimulates insulin secretion and has no other function. (**Ref. 43,** pp. 576–577)

39. (E) All these mechanisms stimulate insulin secretion. The glucose concentration in blood is the most important one. It has a direct effect on the island cells of the pancreas and requires no neuronal or hormonal intermediary. When the level of blood glucose drops, insulin production is decreased as well. Certain amino acids also stimulate insulin production. When the amino acid concentration in blood increases after a protein-rich meal, insulin production increases and the uptake of amino acids by muscle and other cells is promoted. Among the hormones regulating insulin production, the glucose-dependent insulinotropic peptide (GIP) plays an interesting role. The hormone originates in the GI tract and is released on eating. Thus, insulin production is stimulated before the glucose levels rise in the blood. This is referred to as an "anticipatory" component of glucose regulation.

Another anticipatory mechanism is mediated by the parasympathetic fibers going to the pancreas. These are also activated by eating and increase insulin production. (**Ref. 43**, pp. 611–612)

40. (**D**) In most areas glucagon works in direct opposition to insulin. Its major effects are all on the liver, where it binds to the receptors of the plasma membrane of the hepatocytes. This activates adenyl cyclase and generates cyclic AMP. This, in turn, activates cAMP-dependent protein kinase, which phosphorylates the enzyme that mediates the effects of glucagon.

    The effects of glucagon are to increase glycogen breakdown, increase gluconeogenesis, and synthesize ketones. There is only one area in which glucagon and insulin activity follows a parallel course. Both glucagon and insulin production is stimulated by a rise in plasma amino acid concentration. The rise is more significant for insulin, however, than it is for glucagon. (**Ref. 43**, pp. 613–614)

41. (**E**) Cholesterol is carried in the plasma in a variety of lipoprotein combinations. These include the chylomicrons, VLDL (very low-density lipoprotein), and HDL (high-density lipoprotein). The LDLs are the primary carriers and deliver cholesterol from the liver to the cells. HDL takes cholesterol from the tissues and carries it to the liver from which it is excreted in the bile. In common parlance LDL is the "bad" cholesterol which causes atherosclerosis and HDL is "good" cholesterol. In view of this, the diagnostic and prognostic value in plasma cholesterol determination lies not with the total cholesterol levels but with the ratio of LDL to HDL. The lower this ratio, the lower the risk of developing coronary artery disease. (**Ref. 43**, p. 622)

42. (**A**) Growth hormone is secreted by the anterior pituitary. It has probably very little, if any, effect on fetal development. Its primary role is to stimulate cell division in a number of target tissues, such as bone. The effects of the growth hormone on the cells is not direct but is mediated through a messenger that is produced under the stimulation of the growth hormone. This messenger is the insulin-like growth factor, 1 (IGF-1), which used to be

known as somatomedin C. IGF-1 is secreted by the liver and by many other cells.

Lack of growth hormone (dwarfism) may be due to a lack of growth hormone, to a lack of IGF-1, or to the failure of the target cells to respond to IGF-1.

The production of the growth hormone itself is under the control of the hypothalamic hypophysiotropic hormone GHRH (growth hormone-releasing hormone). (**Ref. 43,** pp. 626–627)

43. **(A)** The primary function of TH is the determination of the basal metabolic rate (BMR), that is, the rate at which heat is produced during the basic, resting metabolic state. It increases oxygen consumption and heat production in all systems except the brain. Its absence during the fetal period leads to cretinism. It facilitates both the production and the response to growth hormone and thus is required for the normal growth and development of childhood. It is also required for normal alertness and active reflexes. Significant hypoavailability leads to lethargy, one of the cardinal features of myxedema. It facilitates the sympathetic nervous system and hence tachycardia is one of the diagnostic features of thyrotoxicosis. (**Ref. 43,** p. 632)

44. **(C)** Heat production is primarily a function of muscle activity. Shivering, an oscillating, rhythmical muscle tremor, occurring at a rate of 10–20/sec is the mechanism whereby this is accomplished. The internal heat production is referred to as "shivering thermogenesis." Shivering is the response to external cold but may also occur after the ingestion of large volumes of chilled liquids or ice cream.

There is another mechanism, "non-shivering thermogenesis" in which metabolic rate is increased as a result of increased production of epinephrine and, perhaps, TH as well. In adult humans its role is minimal, although it is a significant component of heat production in infants and some animals. (**Ref. 43,** pp. 639–640)

3
Pharmacology

DIRECTIONS (Questions 45–55): Each of the questions or incomplete statements below is followed by five suggested answers or completions. Select the **one** that is best in each case.

45. Both diazepam and lorazepam
    A. depress respiration
    B. can produce general anesthesia
    C. may produce paradoxical effects (e.g., anxiety and agitation)
    D. are analgesics
    E. have a half-life of 15 to 25 hours

46. Induced emesis and gastric lavage is contraindicated if the ingested poison was
    A. a barbiturate
    B. an opiate
    C. a nonsteroidal anti-inflammatory drug
    D. a drain cleaner
    E. a pesticide

47. Which of the following narcotics is contraindicated in patients with concurrent monoamine oxidase (MAO) inhibitor therapy?
   A. morphine
   B. meperidine
   C. codeine
   D. pentazocine
   E. fentanyl

48. The most important biotransformation responsible for the termination of biological activity of the more lipid-soluble barbiturates is
   A. N-hydroxylation
   B. oxidation of the radicals at C-5
   C. hydrolysis of the barbiturate ring
   D. N-dealkylation
   E. N-glucosylation

49. Which of the following frequently used cardiac drugs may cause severe pulmonary complications?
   A. timolol
   B. propranolol
   C. flecainide
   D. amiodarone
   E. diltiazem

50. A patient receives echothiophate eyedrops for wide-angle glaucoma. Which of the following agents should be avoided in giving general anesthesia?
   A. etomidate
   B. atracurium
   C. propofol
   D. vecuronium
   E. succinylcholine

51. The isozyme known as cytochrome P_{450} plays an important role in biotransformation. Which of the following drugs inhibits P_{450}?
   A. ranitidine
   B. sucralfate
   C. pentagastrin
   D. morphine
   E. cimetidine

52. One of the following anesthetic drugs must be avoided in patients with acute intermittent porphyria or variegated porphyria.
    A. succinylcholine
    B. atracurium
    C. propofol
    D. thiopental
    E. halothane

53. When heparin is used as an anticoagulant, its primary activity is to
    A. decrease platelet aggregation
    B. increase platelet aggregation
    C. increase the rate of the thrombin–antithrombin reaction
    D. decrease the rate of the thrombin–antithrombin reaction
    E. directly inhibit factor VIIa

54. The risk of hemorrhage in patients taking oral anticoagulants is enhanced by
    A. barbiturates
    B. rifampin
    C. phenytoin
    D. acute alcohol intake
    E. pregnancy

55. Which of the following receptor sites is primarily responsible for the analgesic effects of morphine and other potent analgesics?
    A. alpha
    B. delta
    C. kappa
    D. lambda
    E. mu

DIRECTIONS (Questions 56–65): For each of the questions or incomplete statements below, **one** or **more** of the answers given is correct. Select
- **A.** if only 1, 2, and 3 are correct
- **B.** if only 1 and 3 are correct
- **C.** if only 2 and 4 are correct
- **D.** if only 4 is correct
- **E.** if all are correct

56. The complications of oral anticoagulants include
    1. hemorrhage
    2. birth defects
    3. skin necrosis
    4. purple toes

57. The anticholinesterase drugs include
    1. pralidoxime
    2. edrophonium
    3. pilocarpine
    4. pyridostigmine

58. Primary drugs effective in producing deliberate hypotension include
    1. nitroglycerin
    2. sodium nitroprusside
    3. pentolinium
    4. esmolol

59. The so-called high-ceiling diuretics include
    1. acetazolamide
    2. hydrochlorothiazide
    3. spironolactone
    4. ethacrynic acid

60. The withdrawal symptoms in opioid-dependent patients include
    1. sneezing, lacrimation, and coryza
    2. chilliness and pilomotor activity
    3. intestinal spasms and diarrhea
    4. tonic-clonic convulsions

61. Successful drug-free recovery from controlled substance abuse must include
1. inpatient and step-down residential therapy
2. personalized psychotherapy
3. reentry contract
4. methadone therapy

62. Bleomycin
1. causes considerable bone marrow depression
2. cannot be combined with vinblastine
3. is effective only in the treatment of testicular carcinomas
4. causes pulmonary fibrosis and increases O_2 toxicity

63. Esmolol
1. is a selective β_1 antagonist
2. has little if any intrinsic sympathomimetic activity
3. has a short duration of action
4. has its peak hemodynamic effect in 6 to 10 minutes

64. When administering disulfiram to a person who has recently ingested alcoholic beverages, which of the following may be expected?
1. no obvious reaction
2. flushed (scarlet) facies
3. marked hypertension
4. headache, nausea, vomiting, and vertigo

65. The most important parameter(s) in determining the dosage of a drug is (are)
1. clearance
2. volume of distribution
3. bioavailability
4. rates of availability

Pharmacology

Answers and Discussion

The authors have made every effort to thoroughly verify the answers to the questions that appear on the preceding pages. As in any text, however, some inaccuracies and ambiguities may occur. If in doubt, please consult the indicated reference. When no page number(s) are cited, the reference is to a journal article or to a refresher course lecture that should be read in its entirety.

The Editors

45. (C) The benzodiazepines affect most parts of the CNS. They are primarily sedatives and hypnotics although they are used also as anticonvulsants, antianxiety agents, skeletal muscle relaxants, and, in anesthesiology, for premedication and as a supplement to general anesthesia. Except in very large doses they do not depress respiration, and death from benzodiazepines alone is very rare. They do not produce anesthesia. Their effect on circulation is minor, although in doses used for premedication they may produce some hypotension and tachycardia. The benzodiazepines may produce a number of untoward (paradoxical) responses, such as nightmares, anxiety, restlessness, euphoria, hallucinations, suicidal ideation, and hypomanic behavior. The paradoxical reactions are rare but unpredictable.

The benzodiazepines have widely varying half-lives. Diazepam has a half-life of 30 to 60 hours and lorazepam has a half-life of 10 to 20 hours. (**Ref. 15,** pp. 354–356)

46. (D) Induced vomiting and/or gastric lavage is the treatment of choice in most drug or chemical intoxications, except when the ingested substance was (1) corrosive, (2) a CNS stimulant, or (3) a petroleum distillate. In these cases induced vomiting aggravates the damage and may make a relatively mild problem into a much more serious one.

For gastric lavage the largest suitable tube should be used. In comatose patients or in patients who are convulsing, gastric lavage should *never* be attempted unless the airway is first protected by the insertion of a cuffed endotracheal tube. Lavage in the presence of an unprotected airway is, ipso facto, malpractice, and the aspiration likely to occur will be extremely costly to both the patient and the physician. The same rule applies to induced vomiting, particularly if apomorphine is used as the emetic agent. It should also be remembered that apomorphine is a respiratory depressant and therefore should not be used in patients who suffer from a CNS depressant overdose. (**Ref. 15,** pp. 56–57)

47. (B) Patients receiving monoamine oxidase inhibitors (e.g., tranylcypromine) may very rapidly develop a hypertensive crisis and hyperpyrexia when exposed to certain foods or drugs. Meperidine is the only opiate that has this effect, but any food that contains a pressor amine or a substance that can liberate stored catecholamines can trigger this very dangerous reaction. The foods particularly implicated include certain strong cheeses, beer, certain wines, chicken livers, coffee, citrus fruit, chocolate, and canned figs. The hypertensive crisis may be severe enough to cause intracranial hemorrhage and death. (**Ref. 15,** pp. 416–417)

48. (B) For the less lipid-soluble barbiturates, like phenobarbital, N-glucosylation is a major metabolic pathway. The more lipid-soluble ones undergo oxidation of the radicals at C-5, and this oxidation produces alcohols, ketones, phenols, and carbolic acid. These may either appear in the urine in this form or may become conjugated with glucuronic acid. The thiobarbiturates are desulfurated. Only phenobarbital and aprobarbital appear in the urine unchanged to any significant degree. Almost all aprobarbital and

25% of phenobarbital appear in the urine unchanged. The metabolic elimination of the barbiturates is slow, and all the more commonly used hypnotics have a half-life in excess of 24 hours. This makes daily use cumulative and may lead to overdose and abuse. (**Ref. 15,** p. 361)

49. (D) Amiodarone causes a large number of complications, particularly if it is administered over a long period. The complications escalate rapidly after 12 months of treatment and may affect several organ systems. Ten to 15% of the patients develop symptoms of pulmonary fibrosis, and in the patients who do develop this complication, there is a mortality rate of 10%. Other complications of amiodarone include hypo- and hyperthyroidism, cutaneous photosensitivity, corneal microdeposits, and hepatic injury. In about 2% to 5% of the patients on amiodarone, the arrhythmias for which the drug was administered become worse. (**Ref. 15,** p. 868)

50. (E) Echothiophate, a potent and long-acting anticholinesterase, used in the form of eyedrops in the management of glaucoma, does not stay in the conjunctival sac but is absorbed systemically and therefore affects the behavior of certain other drugs. It prolongs the muscle relaxant effects of succinylcholine, and it also prolongs the effects of the ester-linkage local anesthetic agents. Many patients do not think of eyedrops or nose drops as drugs and therefore may omit them when queried about medication use. Patients must be asked specifically about eyedrops and nose drops as part of a standard preanesthetic workup. (**Ref. 15,** p. 144)

51. (E) Cimetidine is the only H_2 blocker that inhibits cytochrome P_{450}. This, in turn, slows the metabolic degradation of a number of drugs and thus prolongs and/or accentuates their effects. The most important drugs whose effects are thus prolonged are warfarin, theophylline, propranolol, nifedipine, quinidine, the tricyclic antidepressants, and some benzodiazepines. In view of this interaction, when cimetidine is prescribed as a continuing medication, other concurrent medications must be revised or switched to some unaffected substitute. When both drugs have to be continued, the dosage of the non-H_2 antagonist may have to be reduced.

H_2 blockers may affect the absorption of certain drugs by changing the acidity of the gastric juice. (**Ref. 15,** p. 901)

52. (D) Among the various porphyrias only the acute intermittent and variegated forms are of great concern to the anesthesiologist. Acute intermittent porphyria is an inborn error of metabolism that affects porphyrin synthesis. Porphyrin synthesis is needed for the production of heme, and this process is catalyzed by the enzyme aminolevulinic acid (ALA). The disease is characterized by acute intermittent attacks of abdominal pain, psychotic behavior, tachycardia, hypertension, peripheral nerve pains, and paresis. This complex syndrome, or some component thereof, can be triggered acutely by certain drugs and drug groups. Most notoriously, the barbiturates are responsible for such attacks, but etomidate, pentazocine, and steroids will also cause them. Ketamine and the benzodiazepines have also been implicated, and even though the evidence is tenuous, these drugs are best avoided. Propofol, the opiates, and inhalational agents are safe. (**Ref. 41**, pp. 375–377)

53. (C) Antithrombin inhibits thrombin only in the presence of heparin. It is the inhibition of thrombin and of factor Xa that accounts for the anticoagulant activity of heparin. The thrombin–antithrombin reaction is enormously accelerated by heparin (1,000×).

In large doses, heparin does interfere with platelet aggregation and prolongs bleeding time. Another, very interesting effect of heparin is the "clearing" of lipemic plasma. It accomplishes this by releasing a lipoprotein lipase, which hydrolyses the circulating triglycerides. After heparin infusion is discontinued, a rebound hyperlipidemia may ensue. (**Ref. 15**, pp. 1314–1315)

54. (D) A number of drugs increase the risk of hemorrhage in patients on oral anticoagulants. These include phenylbutazone, metronidazole, disulfiram, allopurinol, cimetidine, amiodarone, and ethanol. A relative vitamin K deficiency due to dietary or intestinal problems also increases the risk of hemorrhage. Hepatic dysfunction, congestive heart failure, and hypermetabolic states also represent an increased risk. Advancing age also tends to increase the sensitivity of the patient to oral anticoagulants. (**Ref. 15**, pp. 1319–1320)

55. (E) Morphine has ten times the affinity for the mu receptor than for the delta or kappa. (There are no alpha and lambda opiate receptors.) Sufentanyl has 200 times more affinity for the mu receptor than for the other two. This is generally true for all the straight agonist analgesics. The agonist–antagonist analgesics, such as pentazocine, have affinity for the kappa receptors only. These drugs are well known to produce serious psychotomimetic reactions that are not antagonized by naloxone. The reactions may be mediated through the sigma receptors, which also have an affinity for PCP. All three major receptors exert an inhibitory regulation on synaptic transmission, both in the CNS and also in the myenteric plexus. They also all seem to be coupled to guanidine nucleotide binding regulatory proteins, the so-called G proteins. The exact mechanism whereby these couplings regulate ionic flow (K^+ and Ca^{++}) across the respective channels is not clear. (**Ref. 15,** p. 488)

56. **(E)** All of these are potential complications of oral anticoagulant therapy. Hemorrhage is clearly the major toxicity and may lead to death if the hemorrhage occurs in the CNS. Gastrointestinal and renal hemorrhage may also have very serious consequences. The incidence of intracranial hemorrhage is increased by a factor of ten in patients over the age of 50 who are on long-term oral anticoagulant therapy.

    If pregnant women are given oral anticoagulants, abortion or congenital defects may occur. These are not limited to the first trimester, and CNS damage in the newborn has been reported after second and third trimester therapy with warfarin.

    Skin necrosis is a rare but serious complication, frequently requiring debridement and even amputation. The purple toe syndrome consists of a blue discoloration of the toes. Other toxic reactions include diarrhea, cramps, alopecia, dermatitis, fever, and anorexia. (**Ref. 15,** pp. 1320–1321)

57. **(C)** Edrophonium and pyridostigmine, as well as neostigmine and echothiophate, are anticholinesterase drugs that have wide clinical applications in a variety of conditions. They are used in cases of atony of smooth muscle, glaucoma, myasthenia gravis, and to counteract the neuromuscular blocking agents. Pralidoxime, in larger doses, reactivates acetylcholine esterase. Pilocarpine is a cholinomimetic agent and is used primarily in the treatment of wide-angle glaucoma. Physostigmine is useful in counteracting the undesirable effects of atropine and scopolamine and is also very helpful in cases of phenothiazine and tricyclic an-

tidepressant overdoses. It has also been used in the management of Friedreich's ataxia. (**Ref. 15,** pp. 128, 142)

58. **(A)** Sodium nitroprusside and nitroglycerin are the agents of choice in deliberate, controlled hypotension, in order to minimize blood loss during anesthesia for certain surgical procedures. Both can be given as an intravenous infusion, and their effects are sufficiently short-acting so that termination of the infusion will rapidly restore preinfusion blood pressures. Sodium nitroprusside is unstable in solution and must be protected from bright lights. If used for a long period, it may produce increased bleeding by interfering with the clotting mechanism. Nitroprusside can be converted in the body to cyanide and thiocyanate. This reaction can be blocked by the administration of sodium thiosulfate, which will not decrease the vasodilator activity of the nitroprusside. Esmolol or propranolol are frequently used in combination with the more active hypotensive agents, in their role as beta-blockers, to prevent the tachycardia that may negate, at least to some extent, the deliberate hypotension.

    Pentolinium is an excellent hypotensive agent but is not currently available in the United States. (**Ref. 15,** pp. 770, 804)

59. **(D)** Ethacrynic acid and furosemide are the two very potent high-ceiling diuretics that act primarily by preventing the reabsorption of electrolytes in the ascending limb of Henle's loop. Their onset of action is very rapid and diuresis will ensue within minutes. They cause the excretion of sodium, potassium, magnesium, and calcium. Acetazolamide is a carbonic anhydrase inhibitor that acts by inhibiting the excretion of hydrogen ions in the renal tubules. Consequently, the volume of urine produced is alkaline and the excretion of bicarbonates is increased.

    Hydrochlorothiazide is a benzthiazide that acts directly on the excretion of sodium chloride and water. Although it does increase the excretion of potassium, in long-range therapy it is more sparing of potassium than the high-ceiling diuretics.

    Spironolactone is an aldosterone antagonist. It is used primarily in the management of hypertension and in refractory edema. It produces hypokalemia and may produce gynecomastia. (**Ref. 15,** pp. 713 et seq.)

Answers and Discussion: 58–62 / 39

60. (A) The withdrawal symptoms that follow the sudden cessation, or the pharmacologic reversal, of narcotic administration in persons who have developed physical dependence is quite similar, regardless of which narcotic substance had been abused. An exception to this rule is provided by meperidine. The meperidine abstinence syndrome has a more rapid onset, is of shorter duration, and is milder as far as the autonomic signs are concerned. Muscle twitching and restlessness, however, tend to be considerably worse than for the other opiates.

Morphine and heroin abstinence syndrome starts after 8 to 12 hours and peaks at 48 to 72 hours. The patient will be intensely uncomfortable, but the abstinence syndrome is not life threatening. Seizures are practically unknown in these patients.

The barbiturate abstinence syndrome, although similar in many of its manifestations to the opiate abstinence syndrome, is much more severe. Single or multiple seizures and even status epilepticus are not uncommon and may rapidly become life threatening. (**Ref. 15,** pp. 534, 537)

61. (B) The critical feature in recovering from controlled substance abuse is intensive inpatient and residential stepdown unit therapy of at least 90 days' duration. This must be followed by a reentry contract, which specifies regular attendance at AA or NA meetings, initially five times per week and later at least 3 to 4 times per week. The reentry contract also provides for random urine and/or blood testing and continuing contact with an expert addictionologist specializing in the care of the impaired health professional.

Personalized psychotherapy has been helpful in isolated instances, but is generally disappointing. Methadone and buprenorphine therapy has been used with some success, particularly in the United Kingdom (UK), but in health professionals the best and most lasting recovery process was achieved without narcotic replacement therapy. Short therapy courses (28 days) or outpatient management of the impaired physician has proven very unsatisfactory in the large majority of cases. (**Ref. 15,** pp. 563–567 and the author's experience)

62. (D) Bleomycin used clinically is a mixture of bleomycin A_2 and bleomycin B_2. Its primary usefulness is in the treatment of testicular carcinomas, but it is also quite effective against squamous cell carcinomas of the head, neck, and lungs. It has only minimal bone marrow depressant activity, and in this it differs from most other antineoplastic drugs. It can be readily combined with vinblastine and this raises its effectiveness from 30% to 90%. Its primary toxicity affects the skin and the lungs. It causes erythematous, ulcerating lesions over the pressure areas of the body. The most serious complication of bleomycin therapy is the pulmonary toxicity that may progress to fatal pulmonary fibrosis. Bleomycin sensitizes the lungs to oxygen, and exposure to an FiO_2 of more than room air may lead to the dramatic onset of an ARDS-like syndrome, which in some cases may be fatal. This may occur even in patients who had bleomycin therapy many months previously and who had no overt pulmonary symptoms. (**Ref. 15,** pp. 1245–1246)

63. **(E)** Esmolol is a very rapidly acting β_1 blocker. In this regard it differs from propranolol and labetalol, which are nonselective β blockers. It also differs from pindolol in that it has little or no intrinsic sympathomimetic activity. It is particularly useful in the control of supraventricular tachycardias during general anesthesia. It may cause profound hypotension in nonhypertensive patients. The mechanism of this hypotensive effect has not been elucidated. (**Ref. 15,** p. 237)

64. **(C)** Disulfiram is an antioxidant and used as such in industry. It has no appreciable effect on the abstinent person but causes a dramatic syndrome, known as the aldehyde syndrome, in persons who have taken an alcoholic beverage shortly before or after the ingestion of disulfiram. The response is very rapid and consists of flushing, headache, nausea, vomiting, vertigo, hypotension, orthostatic syncope, blurred vision, and confusion. All these symptoms can be attributed to a sharp increase in the acetaldehyde concentration in the body. In fact, the same syndrome can be produced by the infusion of acetaldehyde. Acetaldehyde is a normal metabolic product of ethyl alcohol, and disulfiram works by irreversibly blocking the enzyme aldehyde dehydrogenase. Disulfiram is used effectively in assisting recovering alcoholics who are seriously trying to regain and maintain sobriety. (**Ref. 15,** p. 378)

65. **(A)** Clearance, volume of distribution, and bioavailability are the three cardinal parameters. Clearance is the most important factor in long-range therapy, since the purpose of therapy is a

steady state of the drug in the body. This is a function of intake and clearance. Clearance can be hepatic, renal, pulmonary, gastrointestinal, and so on. The volume of distribution relates the amount of drug in the body to the plasma concentration. There are several ways of calculating it, the simplest being the assumption that the body is a single, uniform compartment. Half-life is one of the measures used in calculating dosage. Clinically useful half-life figures are available for most drugs. From a scientific perspective these times are grossly inaccurate. The third important parameter is bioavailability. It is the fraction of an ingested or otherwise administered substance that ultimately reaches the bloodstream for systemic distribution. There are many components of bioavailability. These include the rate of absorption, first pass elimination in the liver, protein binding, and others. (**Ref. 15, pp. 20–29**)

4
Biochemistry

DIRECTIONS (Questions 66–82): Each of the questions or incomplete statements below is followed by five suggested answers or completions. Select the **one** that is best in each case.

---

66. As a neurotransmitter, norepinephrine
    A. is synthesized from tyrosine
    B. is synthesized primarily in nerve endings of the preganglionic neurons of the sympathetic nervous system
    C. is stored in the adrenal cortex
    D. action is terminated primarily by metabolism by monoamine oxidase
    E. is synthesized from thyroxine

67. Acetylcholine as a neurotransmitter
    A. is metabolized in the liver by acetylcholinesterase
    B. is synthesized in the cytoplasm of the preganglionic and postganglionic sympathetic nerve endings
    C. is synthesized in the cytoplasm of the preganglionic and postganglionic parasympathetic nerve endings
    D. has prolonged activity in patients with atypical pseudocholinesterase
    E. activates only the parasympathetic nervous system

68. Abnormal platelet function
   A. can be corrected by the administration of fresh frozen plasma
   B. is always seen when the platelet count is less than 100,000 cells/mm^3
   C. will result in prolonged PTT and PT coagulation tests
   D. is best measured by the performance of a bleeding time
   E. should be suspected in patients who present with a history of coumadin therapy

69. Aldosterone
   A. is the primary exogenous mineralocorticoid
   B. is synthesized in the adrenal medulla
   C. is secreted in response to renin release by the kidney
   D. promotes renal tubular absorption of potassium to prevent hypokalemia
   E. secretion is increased in response to hyperkalemia

70. Carbon monoxide intoxication
   A. is a result of the lower affinity of hemoglobin for carbon monoxide than for oxygen
   B. results in a shift of the oxyhemoglobin dissociation curve to the right
   C. results in low arterial oxygen saturation in the presence of a normal PaO$_2$
   D. results in an increase in minute ventilation
   E. results in a marked metabolic alkalosis

71. Patients with sickle cell anemia have an increased tendency for their red cells to sickle as a result of
   A. the presence of RBCs containing small amounts of hemoglobin S (HbS)
   B. because oxygen is easily removed from their red cells as the oxyhemoglobin dissociation curve is shifted to the left
   C. because HbS molecules devoid of oxygen tend to stick together and result in abnormal cell shape
   D. the decreased viscosity of abnormal red blood cells
   E. vascular occlusion of small arterioles and capillaries

72. The element zinc is widely distributed in the body and is an important factor in
   A. maintaining the integrity of the extrinsic clotting pathway
   B. establishing the resting membrane potential of cardiac muscle
   C. the proper functioning of the enzyme carbonic anhydrase
   D. the treatment of manic depression
   E. oxygen transport in severely anemic patients

73. The cation magnesium
   A. is second only to potassium as the most abundant extracellular cation
   B. is found almost exclusively in the intracellular fluid
   C. can easily be measured in its ionized form
   D. is not lost in clinical situations in which calcium or sodium is lost from abnormal renal excretion
   E. is stored mostly in muscle tissue

74. The "second messenger" concept in hormonal activity involves the binding of the "first messenger" to the receptor site and the stimulation of which enzyme to catalyze the conversion of ATP to cyclic adenosine monophosphate (cAMP)?
   A. phosphodiesterase
   B. protein kinase
   C. 3′–5′ cyclic adenylic kinase
   D. adenosine 3′–5′ monophosphate
   E. adenyl cyclase

75. The metabolism of cyclic adenosine monophosphate (cAMP) is controlled by the which of the following?
   A. phosphorylase kinase
   B. protein kinase
   C. phosphorylase a
   D. phosphodiesterase
   E. phosphorylase b

76. Branched-chain amino acids are important elements in total parenteral nutrition. Which of the following is a branched-chain amino acid?
   A. cysteine
   B. tryptophan

C. glutamic acid
D. threonine
E. leucine

77. One of the major biochemical differences between RNA and DNA is
    A. the presence of uracil rather than adenine as a pyrimidine base in RNA
    B. ribose as the carbohydrate moiety in RNA; deoxyribose as the carbohydrate in DNA
    C. the use of the different purine base residues in both DNA and RNA
    D. DNA is single- or double-stranded; RNA is double-stranded only
    E. RNA is a strong base, and DNA is a strong acid

78. The oxygen saturation measured by pulse oximetry is not the same as the oxygen saturation measured by laboratory co-oximetry because
    A. pulse oximeters need frequent calibration
    B. pulse oximeters measure "fractional saturation" of all types of hemoglobin
    C. pulse oximeters measure the "functional saturation" of reduced and saturated hemoglobin
    D. pulse oximeters amplify weak signals until a value can be obtained
    E. pulse oximeter sensors are frequently misapplied and give false measurements

79. Patients with liver cirrhosis and portal hypertension usually have a shift of the oxyhemoglobin curve
    A. to the left secondary to decreased 2–3 DPG
    B. to the right secondary to increased 2–3 DPG
    C. no change
    D. lower slope secondary to anemia
    E. increased slope secondary to anemia

80. The treatment of primary hyperuricemia is
    A. by the administration of drugs that block the synthesis of oxypurinol
    B. by the administration of drugs inhibiting xanthine oxidase
    C. by the administration of colchicine to promote renal excretion of uric acid
    D. by the administration of large doses of loop diuretics
    E. by the administration of aspirin

81. The neurotransmitter gamma aminobutyric acid (GABA)
    A. is synthesized in a multistep process with several amino acid precursors
    B. is synthesized from the decarboxylation of glycine
    C. is synthesized as the final product of catecholamine metabolism
    D. is synthesized in a one-step decarboxylation from the amino acid glutamate
    E. is a naturally occurring neurotransmitter

82. The neurotransmitter acetylcholine
    A. is deactivated very slowly once it is released and thus results in increased nerve transmission
    B. degradation is inhibited or blocked by the administration of pseudocholinesterase
    C. degradation is inhibited or blocked by exposure to organofluorophosphates
    D. degradation is inhibited or blocked in patients with myasthenia syndrome
    E. degradation is increased by succinylcholine

DIRECTIONS (Questions 83–110): For each of the questions or incomplete statements below, **one** or **more** of the answers or completions given is correct. Select
- **A.** if only 1, 2, and 3 are correct
- **B.** if only 1 and 3 are correct
- **C.** if only 2 and 4 are correct
- **D.** if only 4 is correct
- **E.** if all are correct

83. Common properties of the biological membranes include the following:
    1. membrane constituents are covalently bonded to each other to give the membrane structure
    2. membrane lipids are amphipathic molecules (i.e., the lipid portion has a predominant hydrophobic surface)
    3. most membrane protein to lipid ratios are close to 50:50
    4. membranes are symmetrical structures

84. The Krebs or citric acid cycle
    1. generates acetyl CoA from pyruvate, which commits carbon atoms from glucose either to oxidation or to incorporation into lipid
    2. is amphibolic (i.e., operates both catabolically and anabolically)
    3. oxidizes the acetyl group of acetyl CoA to two molecules of CO_2, which conserves the liberated free energy for use in ATP generation
    4. is less efficient energetically than the direct oxidation of acetate to CO_2 through gloxylate

85. It is true of immunoglobulins that
    1. they are specific proteins that can recognize and bind to antigens
    2. the antibody fragment Fab is responsible for binding to the antigen
    3. they contain at least two heavy chains and two light chains
    4. their classification is determined by the heavy chain

86. Specific immunoglobulins bind to various cell types. Which of the following is (are) true?
    1. IgG immunoglobulin binds to mast cells, as well as platelets, lymphocytes, and neutrophils
    2. IgM binds only to mast cells
    3. IgE binds to mast cells, basophils, and lymphocytes
    4. both IgM and IgE activate the complement cascade

87. Which of the following is (are) true statement(s) about the extracellular protein collagen?
    1. nearly every third residue is glycine
    2. the enzyme prolyl hydroxylase requires vitamin B_{12} to assure adequate activity
    3. collagen synthesized in the presence of ascorbic acid is very stable
    4. nearly one-third of the amino acid residues are hydroxylsines

88. The augmented release of free fatty acids in the diabetic patient results in
    1. the production of acetone
    2. beta oxidation of these free fatty acids to beta-hydroxybutyric acid
    3. the production of acetoacetic acid
    4. increased production of glucagon

89. Massive blood transfusions may lead to
    1. metabolic acidosis
    2. hypocalcemia
    3. hyperkalemia
    4. decreased P_{50}

90. Vitamin K plays an essential role in the clotting mechanism because
    1. it is water soluble and found only in citrus fruits
    2. it promotes the attachment of clotting factors II, VII, IX, and X to calcium
    3. it has no known syndrome of deficiency
    4. it is synthesized in the gastrointestinal tract

91. Myoglobin
    1. binds half as much oxygen as normal hemoglobin
    2. is a copper-containing pigment

3. has a lesser affinity for oxygen than hemoglobin
4. is found in skeletal muscle

92. Cerebral metabolism
    1. relies on intrinsic stores of glucose
    2. is markedly higher for children
    3. can easily use anaerobic metabolic pathways for energy production
    4. accounts for 15% of cardiac output

93. The termination of action of norepinephrine is accomplished by
    1. reuptake into the presynaptic terminals
    2. extraneural uptake
    3. metabolism by MAO and COMT
    4. diffusion

94. Which of the following are purine derivatives?
    1. adenine
    2. uracil
    3. guanine
    4. cytosine

95. Methemoglobin, HbA, is a functional abnormality of a red blood cell that
    1. results from the iron in heme being in the ferrous state
    2. results in a shift of the oxyhemoglobin curve to the left
    3. is diagnosed by the presence of normal SaO_2 and low PaO_2
    4. is kept below 1% of total hemoglobin by the enzyme methemoglobin reductase

96. Concerning endorphins,
    1. they are found in areas with high concentrations of opioid receptors
    2. the posterior pituitary contains the peptides that are the precursors of the specific endorphins
    3. they are inhibitory for the neurons that release neurotransmitters for pain
    4. they are not found in the spinal cord area

50 / 4: Biochemistry

97. Oxidative phosphorylation
  1. occurs only in the mitochondria of the cell
  2. is controlled by pyruvate dehydrogenase, which is inhibited by high levels of NADH, GTP, and acetyl CoA
  3. results in the production of up to 38 moles of ATP
  4. can occur both with or without oxygen

98. Cholesterol
  1. is found entirely in plasma within lipoprotein complexes
  2. is a precursor for the synthesis of corticosteroids, estradiol, and testosterone
  3. endogenous production is increased when exogenous cholesterol intake is decreased
  4. contains very high concentrations of fatty acids

99. Lipoproteins
  1. are synthesized in the liver
  2. are composed of cholesterol, triglycerides, and proteins
  3. function to provide a transport mechanism of lipids in and out of specific target tissues
  4. high-density lipoprotein (HDL) provides for the transport of most of the cholesterol in the body

100. Many of the amino acids are synthesized from intermediates of the citric acid cycle. Choose the correct precursor and the amino acid synthesized.
  1. pyruvate/alanine
  2. oxaloacetate/aspartate
  3. alpha ketoglutarate/glutamine
  4. phosphoenolpyruvate/tyrosine

101. Glutathione is a tripeptide that participates in a variety of processes. Which of the following (is) are true?
  1. provides a passive transport mechanism for amino acids to pass through cell membranes
  2. reacts with peroxides to form water
  3. reacts with peroxides to form glutamic acid
  4. provides an energy-driven transport of amino acids into cells

102. Concerning the metabolism of hemoglobin
 1. the cleavage of the A and B rings and the removal of the iron molecule results in the formation of biliverdin
 2. the bridge between the C and D rings of biliverdin is reduced to form bilirubin
 3. globin is reduced to its component amino acids
 4. carbon dioxide is released by the oxidative cleavage of the A and B rings

103. Blood glucose levels are controlled by
 1. the secretion of glucagon by pancreatic cells results from low blood glucose
 2. the stimulation of glycogen synthesis in the liver by insulin secretion
 3. the increased rate of glucose transport across cell membranes in response to insulin secretion
 4. the stimulation of gluconeogenesis in the liver by epinephrine and norepinephrine

104. Which of the following antibiotics inhibit(s) protein synthesis?
 1. tetracycline
 2. erythromycin
 3. chloramphenicol
 4. penicillin

105. The mechanism by which fibrin forms a stable clot involves which of the following?
 1. fibrinogen cleavage by thrombin to form fibrinopeptides
 2. the attraction of opposite charged portions of the fibrinopeptides
 3. stabilization of the clot by fibrin-stabilizing factor XIIIa
 4. the release of very large amounts of tissue thromboplastin, which will yield molecule for molecule amounts of fibrin

106. The oxidation of fatty acids
 1. occurs in the endoplasmic reticulum or in the mitochondria
 2. requires the transport of the fatty acid across the mitochondrial membrane
 3. produces large amounts of metabolic energy
 4. produces small amounts of metabolic energy compared to glucose metabolism

52 / 4: Biochemistry

107. The biochemical structures known as protoporphyrins include
    1. chlorophyll
    2. hemoglobin
    3. cytochromes
    4. mitochondria

108. The sodium–potassium pump (NA^+-K^+ pump) is catalyzed by Na^+-K^+-ATPase. Which of the following is true concerning this transport system?
    1. it provides for the electrical excitability of nerve cells
    2. it provides the free energy for active transport of glucose into some cells
    3. it provides for the control of intracellular water
    4. it is inhibited by cardiac glycosides

109. The regulation of the calcium (Ca^+) pump is controlled by
    1. the level of free ATP in the cytosol
    2. through the mediation of calmodulin (CaM)
    3. the activation of the Na^+-K^+-ATPase
    4. the amount of intracellular calcium

110. Prostaglandins are eicosanoid hormones. They
    1. are synthesized from arachidonic acid
    2. mediate the inflammatory response
    3. are inhibited by aspirin
    4. induce blood clotting

Biochemistry

Answers and Discussion

The authors have made every effort to thoroughly verify the answers to the questions that appear on the preceding pages. As in any text, however, some inaccuracies and ambiguities may occur. If in doubt, please consult the indicated reference. When no page number(s) are cited, the reference is to a journal article or to a refresher course lecture that should be read in its entirety.

The Editors

66. **(A)** Norepinephrine is synthesized from tyrosine via several enzymatic steps involving the formation of precursors DOPA, and dopamine. The site of the synthesis is the cytoplasm of the postganglionic sympathetic nerve ending. Storage sites for norepinephrine include the adrenal medulla, where most of the norepinephrine is converted to epinephrine. The termination of action is most importantly by reuptake into the postganglionic sympathetic nerve endings. Metabolism by MAO is of relatively minor importance in terminating the action of norepinephrine. (**Ref. 41,** pp. 347–352)

67. **(C)** Acetylcholine synthesis occurs in the cytoplasm of postganglionic and preganglionic parasympathetic nerve endings, and when released by the arrival of an action potential it can activate receptors in both the parasympathetic and sympathetic nervous

systems. It is metabolized almost exclusively at its sites of activity by the enzyme acetylcholinesterase to choline for re-uptake back into the parasympathetic nerve endings. The pseudocholinesterase of plasma has essentially no effect on the metabolism of acetylcholine. (**Ref. 41,** pp. 647–650)

68. **(D)** Abnormal platelet function can be best tested by performance of a standardized skin bleeding time. Performance of a PTT and/or PT will not demonstrate prolonged bleeding tendencies because platelets are not required to perform these coagulation tests. Prolonged bleeding usually is not seen until the platelet count is less than 50,000, assuming that the platelets have normal function. Correction of abnormal function of the platelets is by the transfusion of platelets, not FFP, which contains very few if any functioning platelets. Coumadin acts on only factors II, VII, IX, and X, not on platelets. (**Ref. 40,** pp. 409–417)

69. **(C)** Aldosterone is the principal endogenous mineralocorticoid secreted by the adrenal cortex. Its synthesis and release are stimulated not only by hypokalemia but also by angiotensin II as a result of renin release by the kidney. Aldosterone regulates intracellular fluid volume by promoting resorption of sodium from the renal tubules, and it promotes the renal excretion of potassium. (**Ref. 41,** p. 358)

70. **(C)** The diagnosis of carbon monoxide poisoning can be difficult if one relies on pulse oximetry. The symptoms depend on the amount of carboxyhemoglobin present. Exposure to low levels of CO cause irritability and altered visual and motor skills. Severe poisoning results in seizures, coma, respiratory failure, and death. Minute ventilation will not usually change until the development of acidosis from tissue hypoxia, and also because the carotid bodies respond to changes in PaO_2, which is normal in CO intoxication. (**Ref. 40,** p. 536)

71. **(C)** The removal of oxygen from HbS is the cause for the abnormal cell shape. The presence of RBCs containing large amounts of HbS (up to 70% to 98%) is characteristic of sickle cell anemia, small amounts of HbS are characteristic of the sickle cell trait. Blood viscosity is increased in sickle cell anemia by the sickled cells sticking together to form long aggregates known as tactoids, which cause vascular occlusion. (**Ref. 40,** p. 401)

72. (C) Zinc is an important element because it has been identified as being part of more than 120 enzymes including carbonic anhydrase. It also has a pronounced effect on amino acid synthesis and metabolism. It has no function in clotting or cardiac muscle physiology. (**Ref. 22,** pp. 481–482)

73. (B) Magnesium is the second most common intracellular cation, with potassium being the most common one. It cannot be measured by clinical laboratories in its ionized form. Between 50% to 60% of the magnesium is located in the skeletal system, and its excretion and resorption from the kidney follow along with calcium and sodium. (**Ref. 36,** pp. 910–911)

74. (E) The first messenger, a neurotransmitter, binds to the receptor site and stimulates the enzyme adenyl cyclase, which in turn catalyzes the conversion of ATP to cAMP, which will then phosphorylate multiple cellular reactions. The cascade from the first messenger to the effector response also depends upon whether an alpha or beta receptor is stimulated. Activated alpha receptors inhibit the formation of cAMP and bypass the second messenger to get an effector organ response. Activated beta receptors, on the other hand, stimulate adenyl cyclase to convert ATP to cAMP. (**Ref. 7,** pp. 335–336)

75. (D) The formation of cAMP is catalyzed by the enzyme phosphodiesterase. Manipulation of this enzyme by agents that either inhibit or stimulate it acts to control the levels of cAMP. For instance, beta-adrenergic agonists stimulate the formation of cAMP, while alpha-2 agonists inhibit the enzyme adenyl cyclase that leads to less cAMP being formed. Stimulating or blocking this enzyme is also important in the treatment of various conditions such as bronchospasm. (**Ref. 7,** pp. 336–337)

76. (E) The branched-chain amino acids have been shown to have a beneficial effect in states where metabolic stress leads to decreased catabolism. They serve as energy substrates, as well as promoting the synthesis of muscle and visceral protein, and they reduce the breakdown of muscle protein. Examples of the

56 / 4: Biochemistry

branched-chain amino acids are leucine, isoleucine, and valine. (**Ref. 7,** pp. 276–278)

77. **(B)** The presence of uracil rather than thiamine differentiates RNA from DNA. Both RNA and DNA use the same purine base residues, with specific base pairing for DNA. Both nucleotides are moderately strong acids. (**Ref. 44,** pp. 740–743)

78. **(C)** Oxygen saturation measured by pulse oximetry is known as the "functional saturation" of hemoglobin and represents the amount of oxyhemoglobin reported as a percentage of the total of reduced hemoglobin and oxyhemoglobin. (Functional SaO_2 = $(O_2Hb/O_2Hb + $ reduced Hb$) \times 100$.) Laboratory cooximeters use different measurement methods to distinguish other types of Hb and to measure fractional saturation. (Fractional saturation = $O_2Hb/(O_2Hb + $ reduced Hb $+ $ COHb $+ $ MetHb$) \times 100$.) Pulse oximeters are calibrated in the factory. (**Ref. 7,** p. 742)

79. **(B)** The erythrocytes of patients with cirrhosis of the liver and portal hypertension have an increased content of 2–3 DPG, which shifts the oxyhemoglobin curve to the right and reduces the affinity of Hb for oxygen. (**Ref. 7,** p. 1192)

80. **(B)** Treatment of primary hyperuricemia, or gout, is by the administration of allopurinol, which inhibits the action of xanthine oxidase, the enzyme that converts xanthine to uric acid. Colchicine reduces the inflammatory responses to uric acid crystals but does not alter the renal excretion of uric acid. Oxypurinol is an active metabolite of allopurinol. (**Ref. 41,** pp. 260–261)

81. **(D)** GABA is one of the physiologically active amines that are classified as neurotransmitters or hormones. Other examples of these amines include norepinephrine, epinephrine, and dopamine. GABA is synthesized as a one-step process involving the decarboxylation of the amino acid glutamate by glutamate decarboxylase, whereas the other amines are the product of several steps in the tyrosine metabolism. The GABA receptor is also known to be a binding site for barbiturates and benzodiazepines. (**Ref. 44,** pp. 708–710)

82. (C) The organofluorophosphates are of the class of nerve gases used by the military and which irreversibly block the action of the acetylcholinesterases. They are also found in various insecticides. Atropine may be effective in overcoming some of the effects of the acetylcholinesterase blockade. Treatment, however, requires very large doses of atropine, in the range of 35 to 70 μg/kg intravenously every 3 to 10 minutes to overcome the nicotinic muscle paralysis and central respiratory depression. (**Ref. 44,** p. 1168)

83. (B) Biological membranes are asymmetric structures containing lipid and protein, covalently bound to provide structure. Although the protein to lipid ratio varies in different membranes, most membranes are at least 50% protein. Membrane proteins, not lipids, are amphipathic molecules, with the protein segment immersed in the membrane's nonpolar interior with predominantly hydrophobic surface residues, and the portion of the protein that extends into the aqueous environment is sheathed with polar residues. (**Ref. 44,** pp. 284–287)

84. (A) During aerobic metabolism, pyruvate is oxidized to acetyl CoA, which then enters the tricarboxylic acid cycle. Pyruvate must enter the mitochondria and relies on intact mitochondrial function. If pyruvate is not metabolized, as above, it may be converted to lactate, which is a metabolic dead end. The decarboxylation of pyruvate by pyruvate dehydrogenase is irreversible and is the only pathway for the synthesis of acetyl CoA. The process is regulated by acetyl CoA and NADH and by the reversible phosphorylation/dephosphorylation of the pyruvate dehydrogenase. (**Ref. 44,** pp. 506–511)

85. (E) Antibodies are specific proteins known as immunoglobulins. They are composed of at least two heavy chains and two light chains bound together by a disulfide bond. The Fc or crystallizable fragment is responsible for the unique biological property of the different classes of immunoglobulins. (**Ref. 7,** p. 1432)

86. (B) The results of antibody–antigen binding depend upon the cell type that is bound and on the specific type of activation. Understanding the activation of specific cell types is important not only for understanding the mechanisms of allergic reactions but also for their treatment. All but one of the IgG immunoglobulins and IgM activates the complement system. IgM binds only to lymphocytes. (Ref. 7, pp. 1432–1433)

87. (B) Collagen has a very distinctive amino acid composition, with one-third of its residues being glycine and another 15% to 30% being 4-hydroxyproline and proline. The synthesis of collagen requires that ascorbic acid (vitamin C) be present to maintain the active form of the enzyme prolyl hydroxylase. (Ref. 44, p. 160)

88. (A) Due to a lack of insulin, abnormal fat metabolism in the diabetic patient leads to accelerated lipid metabolism and the increased formation of the ketone bodies, acetone, acetoacetic acid, and beta hydroxybutyric acid. These increased free fatty acids have multiple metabolic effects, including interference with carbohydrate phosphorylation in muscle, leading to further hyperglycemia. Glucagon is stimulated in part by hypoglycemia, and increased secretion is not a direct result of hyperglycemia. (Ref. 7, p. 1257)

89. (D) Massive transfusion of stored blood means the administration of increased amounts of potassium, but unless a patient has renal impairment and is prone to hyperkalemia, this is not a problem during transfusion. Likewise, transfusion of banked blood containing citrate does not result in clinically apparent hypocalcemia. The lack of 2–3 diphosphoglycerate in stored blood results in a leftward shift of the oxyhemoglobin dissociation curve and a resultant decrease in the P_{50} that could theoretically result in impaired oxygen transfer. (Ref. 40, pp. 422–424)

90. (C) Vitamin K is a lipid-soluble vitamin found in a wide variety of foods. Deficiency of vitamin K may occur for many reasons, from liver failure or decreased dietary intake to decreased production in the gut. Its function is to convert the glutamic acid residues to gamma-carboxyglutamic acid residues of the above coagulation factors. (Ref. 41, pp. 557–559)

91. (D) Myoglobin is an iron-containing pigmented compound that resembles hemoglobin but that binds only one molecule of oxygen. This oxygen is bound very tightly and will be released only when the PO_2 is very low. Myoglobin is the only reserve supply of oxygen for muscle tissue. (Ref. 41, p. 738)

92. (C) The brain has no glucose stores of its own and relies entirely upon adequate cerebral blood flow to deliver glucose and oxygen for its metabolism. Anaerobic metabolism produces only two ATPs. This is not enough energy substrate to sustain the brain's energy needs; thus, the anaerobic metabolic pathway is not a viable option for maintaining adequate cerebral function. **(Ref. 7,** pp. 872–875)

93. (E) The rapid inactivation of neurotransmitters is extremely important in modulating their end organ effects. The inactivation of catecholamines occurs by three pathways, the major one being the reuptake into the presynaptic terminals for storage and reuse. The other pathways are extraneural uptake and diffusion. Norepinephrine inactivation occurs almost entirely by reuptake into the terminals of the presynaptic neuron, with a small amount being metabolized and then diffused out of the nerve terminal. **(Ref. 7,** p. 329)

94. (B) The nitrogenous bases of the nucleotides are derivatives of either purine or pyrimidine. The major purine components of nucleic acids are adenine and guanine, and the major pyrimidine residues are those of cytosine, uracil, and thymine. **(Ref. 44,** p. 741)

95. (C) Methemoglobin is HbA in which the iron is found in the ferric state and therefore cannot bind reversibly with oxygen. This results in a shift of the oxyhemoglobin curve to the left. Diagnosis is made by the presence of normal PaO_2 and low saturation. The pulse oximeter almost always reads 85% no matter what the PaO_2. **(Ref. 40,** p. 403)

96. (B) Endorphins are specific ligands that can activate opiate receptors in areas of high concentrations of these opioid receptors, such as the central nervous system as well as the spinal cord. It is thought that the precursors dynorphin and beta lipotropin are produced in the anterior pituitary gland and that hydrolysis of these substances gives rise to the endorphins. **(Ref. 41,** pp. 72–73)

97. (E) The process by which glucose is broken down to provide energy is glycolysis and the oxidation of the end products of glycolysis. Glucose splits into two molecules of pyruvate, which enter the mitochondria and eventually undergo oxidative phosphorylation. This reaction proceeds optimally in the presence of adequate amounts of oxygen, but it can also proceed anaerobically for a short time if oxygen is lacking. Carbohydrates are the only nutrients that can form ATP without oxygen. (**Ref. 40,** p. 820)

98. **(A)** Cholesterol does not contain fatty acids, but its nucleus is synthesized from the degradation products of fatty acid molecules, giving it many of the characteristics of lipids. Fatty acids, synthesized in the liver from acetate, may then be converted to triglyceride, esterified with cholesterol, incorporated into phospholipids, or oxidized to CO_2 or ketone bodies. All the cholesterol in plasma is in lipoprotein complexes with the low-density lipoproteins representing the major component. (**Ref. 40,** p. 820)

99. **(A)** Lipoproteins provide not only the structure for cell membranes but are also the basis for the transport of fatty acids for energy production, and hormone synthesis. Most cholesterol is transported via the low-density lipoprotein (LDL), which is taken up by the liver by receptor-mediated endocytosis. (**Ref. 40,** p. 821)

100. **(A)** Both essential and nonessential amino acids are synthesized by pathways that are present only in plants and microorganisms. Many of the essential animo acids must be derived from diet, whereas several nonessential amino acids can be synthesized from the intermediate products of the citric acid cycle. Phosphoenolpyruvate is not an intermediate product of the citric acid cycle. (**Ref. 44,** pp. 713–714)

101. **(C)** Amino acid transport into cells occurs via the synthesis and breakdown of glutathione and requires that the glutathione be transported from the interior portion of the cell to the external surface, where a transfer of a portion of the glutathione molecule to the external amino acid occurs. This altered amino acid then is transported back into the cell via the gamma glutamyl cycle. (**Ref. 44,** pp. 709–712)

102. **(A)** The degradation of hemoglobin is accomplished by the cleavage of the heme ring structure by the enzyme heme oxygenase. This step results in the release of the iron molecule and in

the formation of carbon monoxide (CO), which if it were not for one of the distal residues of heme, would allow the preferential binding of CO instead of oxygen by hemoglobin. Biliverdin and bilirubin are pigmented compounds that give the characteristic coloring to bruises. (**Ref. 44,** pp. 706–708)

103. (B) The response to low blood glucose levels, caused by increased use, is mediated by the hormone glucagon, which is secreted by the pancreatic alpha cells. Glucagon receptors in the liver respond by increasing cAMP, which stimulates the breakdown of glycogen and an eventual increase in blood glucose. Epinephrine and norepinephrine increase glucose levels primarily by their action on muscle tissue. (**Ref. 44,** pp. 476–477)

104. (A) The antibiotics are known ribosomal inhibitors. They are known to inhibit a variety of essential biological processes, including DNA replication, transcription, and, in the majority of situations, blockage of the translation processes in protein metabolism. Penicillin is known to alter bacterial cell wall metabolism, but it does not interfere with protein metabolism per se. (**Ref. 44,** pp. 930–931)

105. (B) The blood-clotting cascade, in which very small amounts of tissue thromboplastin released into the blood yield a very large amount of fibrin, is due to the amplification nature of the clotting mechanism. Fibrinogen does not spontaneously form a stable clot because of the "like" electrical charges of the molecules that repel or prevent aggregation, whereas the fibrinopeptides have dissimilar electrical charges that attract or hold the molecules together. (**Ref. 44,** pp. 1090–1091)

106. (A) The fatty acids must first be catalyzed to form fatty acyl-CoA, which is catalyzed by at least three acyl-CoA synthetases. This then allows the fatty acyl-CoA to be transported to the site of oxidation within the mitochondria. This process of oxidation produces huge amounts of metabolic energy. For example, one molecule of palmitate has a net yield of 129 ATP, compared to a net yield of 2 ATP for the oxidation of glucose. (**Ref. 44,** pp. 621–626)

107. **(A)** The cyclic tetrapyrroles chlorophyll, hemoglobin, and the cytochromes are all derived biosynthetically from protoporphyrin IX. These structures differ in such things as the central metal ion, as well as in their biochemical functions. Chlorophyll is the principal light receptor in plants, and hemoglobin is the principal carrier of oxygen. (**Ref. 44,** p. 589)

108. **(E)** The active transport system of Na^+-K^+-ATPase is multifunctional. The active extrusion of sodium out of the cell, which is accompanied by water, prevents animal cells from swelling. 70% of the ATP produced by cells is used to maintain this pump mechanism. Drugs such as digitalis inhibit this pump and result in increased intracellular sodium. Increased intracellular sodium, in turn, leads to more calcium entering the cell and increased muscle contractility—in this case, of cardiac muscle. (**Ref. 44,** pp. 495–496)

109. **(C)** The regulation of the calcium pump in the plasma membrane is controlled by the levels of calcium mediated by calmodulin. CaM is activated by increased levels of intracellular calcium. CaM, in turn, increases the activity of the Ca^+-ATPase pump, which again leads to decreased intracellular calcium. (**Ref. 44,** pp. 496–497)

110. **(E)** Prostaglandins are the precursors of many related compounds, such as the thromboxanes that are important in blood coagulation. They also regulate the sleep/wake cycle, blood pressure control, and the production of pain and fever. One of the best known blockers of the prostaglandins is aspirin, which inhibits prostaglandin synthesis and alters the ability of the coagulation system to adequately form a stable fibrin clot. (**Ref. 44,** pp. 658–659)

5
Physics, Equipment, and Monitoring

DIRECTIONS (Questions 111–122): Each of the questions or incomplete statements below is followed by five suggested answers or completions. Select the **one** that is best in each case.

111. Microshock is defined as current below
    A. 100 mAmps
    B. 50 mA
    C. 10 mA
    D. 1 mA
    E. 1 µA

112. Unipolar electrocautery uses which of the following?
    A. low-frequency current
    B. direct current (DC)
    C. 60 Hz alternating current (AC)
    D. 500,000 to 1,000,000 Hz alternating current (radio frequencies)
    E. high current density at the return plate

113. X-ray exposure decreases
 A. directly with distance
 B. as the third power of the distance
 C. with back-scattered radiation
 D. below 1 rem
 E. as the square of the distance

114. Properly functioning proportioning systems protect against
 A. wrong supply gas attached to yoke or pipeline
 B. circuit leaks
 C. downstream leaks of gases
 D. inert gas administration
 E. setting of hypoxic mixtures of N_2O/O_2 at the flowmeter

115. The desflurane vaporizer needs unique features, because
 A. desflurane corrodes the materials used in standard vaporizers
 B. desflurane vapor pressure is so low (240 mm Hg)
 C. desflurane vapor pressure is so high (669 mm Hg)
 D. desflurane is very potent (MAC <0.6%)
 E. desflurane is degraded in soda lime

116. The safety features in modern anesthesia machines include all of the following EXCEPT
 A. fluted oxygen flowmeter control
 B. oxygen flowmeter upstream
 C. key-indexed vaporizers
 D. fail-safe valves
 E. vaporizer interlocks

117. Since new anesthesia machines incorporate new design features, the 1992 FDA Anesthesia Apparatus Check-out Recommendations differs from the 1986 version in that
 A. a check is no longer required
 B. a negative pressure suction bulb is required for all machines
 C. vaporizer leaks can no longer be detected
 D. inspection of CO_2 absorbent is added
 E. scavenging system is checked

118. Which of the following is NOT true for a nitrous oxide tank?
  A. color blue
  B. full volume of gas at room temperature and pressure is 1590 liters
  C. pressure at 1590 liters is 725 psi
  D. volume of gas at 362.5 psi is 795 liters
  E. the pressure is at the saturated vapor pressure, or 725 psi

119. Isotopes are atoms
  A. with the same number of neutrons but fewer protons
  B. with the same number of electrons but more or fewer neutrons
  C. with one or more fewer electrons
  D. with one or more additional electrons
  E. with one less proton, but one more neutron

120. Which of the following intravenous catheters would allow the greatest fluid flow, assuming that the inside diameter of the 20, 18, and 16 gauge catheters is 0.8, 1.0, and 1.2 mm respectively?
  A. 1 1/2 -inch 18-gauge catheter
  B. 1 1/2 -inch 20-gauge catheter
  C. 12-inch triple-lumen with three 20-gauge lumens
  D. 6-inch 16-gauge catheter
  E. 2-inch 18-gauge catheter

121. Because oxygen is a gas at room temperature, its response to pressure changes can be predicted by the ideal gas law. If an E-cylinder (volume ≈ 5 liters) shows a pressure of 1000 PSIG (1 atmosphere = 15 PSI), how long will it be able to provide a 2-liter flow?
  A. 30 minutes
  B. 1 hour 45 minutes
  C. 2 hours
  D. 2 hours 45 minutes
  E. 4 hours 15 minutes

122. Over the past decade monitors have been developed to measure respiratory gases and vapors continuously from the airway. The most commonly used measurement methods are infrared absorption, mass spectrometry, and Raman scattering analysis. Monitoring based on Raman scattering and mass spectrometry have been advocated because infrared gas analysis cannot measure the following gases
   A. vapor anesthetics
   B. nitrous oxide
   C. oxygen
   D. nitrogen
   E. oxygen and nitrogen

DIRECTIONS (Questions 123–143): For each of the questions or incomplete answers below, **one** or **more** of the answers or completions are correct. Select
   A. if only 1, 2, and 3 are correct
   B. if only 1 and 3 are correct
   C. if only 2 and 4 are correct
   D. if only 4 is correct
   E. if all are correct

---

123. In a patient with a functioning pacemaker, which of the following would be recommended?
   1. placement of return electrode close to pacemaker generator
   2. use of unipolar cautery
   3. preop placement of an external VVO pacemaker
   4. physical monitoring of pulse amplitude and presence

124. Protection from macroshock is afforded by
   1. grounding the patient
   2. grounding the equipment
   3. nonconductive tubing
   4. the line isolation monitor

125. Which of the following statements are true regarding ventilators?
   1. ascending bellows ventilators ascend during expiration
   2. scavenging does not occur
   3. descending bellows ascend during a disconnect
   4. the driving gas contains nitrous oxide

126. ECG optical isolation involves
   1. power transmission by laser
   2. electrical isolation of the patient
   3. fiberoptic computer cables
   4. isolation of the signal coming from the patient

127. Ion-sensitive electrodes (Na, K, Ca) are based upon which of the following principles?
   1. movement of ions across a selective membrane
   2. the Nernst equation
   3. conversion of a chemical signal to an electrical one
   4. solubility product constant

128. Which of the following are true regarding CO_2 absorbers?
   1. optimal mesh size is between 4 and 8 mesh
   2. volume is less than 1 tidal volume to prevent rebreathing
   3. position of the absorber alters efficiency
   4. all circuits require one

129. Which of the following induce(s) artifact in ECG tracings?
   1. electrocautery
   2. cardiopulmonary bypass pump
   3. 60 Hz power lines
   4. muscle fasciculations

130. To prevent rebreathing of carbon dioxide, which of the following must be true in a circle system with CO_2 absorber?
   1. unidirectional valves between patient and reservoir on both inspiratory and expiratory limbs of circuit
   2. fresh gas flow must not enter between expiratory valve and patient
   3. pop-off cannot be located between patient and inspiratory valve
   4. flows must be greater than minute ventilation

131. Which of the following is (are) true of an E oxygen cylinder in the United States?
   1. full pressure is 1900 psi
   2. volume at 70°F is 660 liters
   3. color is green
   4. color is white

132. A DC defibrillating shock
 1. can polarize ECG electrodes and block them for several seconds
 2. may damage an ECG amplifier unless protected by a diode shunt
 3. may cause skin burns
 4. produces a bidirectional voltage spike

133. The Bain circuit
 1. should be used with a gas scavenging system
 2. is a coaxial modification of the Mapleson D circuit
 3. allows great flexibility in positioning the patient
 4. can be used with flows as low as 250 mL/min

134. Infrared light absorption is used to measure the concentration of a substance dissolved in a clear solution. This principle, known as Beer's Law, is employed in capnometers and pulse oximeters. Increasing light absorption is caused by
 1. increasing the path length of light
 2. increasing the concentration of substance
 3. increasing the number of absorbers
 4. a larger absorption coefficient

135. A study comparing two methods of measuring cardiac output reports that they obtained a correlation coefficient of 0.9. From this result you can assume that
 1. there is a 90% chance the two methods are equal
 2. approximately 10% of the time the two methods will not agree
 3. you may be able to use the two methods interchangeably for clinical purposes
 4. there is a high positive association between the two methods of measurement

136. During the induction of a patient for a craniotomy for tumor removal, the systolic pressure measured by the arterial line is noted to be significantly greater than that measured by the noninvasive oscillometric blood pressure cuff. Which of the following would

increase the "overshoot" of the systolic measurement by the invasive arterial monitoring system?
1. increasing heart rate
2. increasing length of fluid-filled high-pressure tubing
3. increasing diameter of the arterial catheter
4. smaller diameter of the arterial catheter

137. A burn victim is brought to the emergency room with obvious signs of smoke inhalation. A pulse oximeter indicates a saturation level of 99% with the patient breathing supplemental oxygen. The following can be assumed regarding the presence of carbon monoxide poisoning in the patient:
    1. the carboxyhemoglobin level is less than 1%
    2. the carboxyhemoglobin level is greater than 10%
    3. the carboxyhemoglobin level is not of a dangerous range
    4. little conclusion can be drawn regarding carboxyhemoglobin

138. A 64-year-old patient is undergoing a right total hip repair under a general anesthesia. In the middle of the procedure it is noted that the end tidal CO_2 values have dropped from 40 mm Hg to approximately 20 mm Hg over several minutes. An arterial blood gas is drawn and the $PaCO_2$ value is 40 mm Hg. What can be concluded from these data?
    1. either the blood gas machine or the capnometer is in error
    2. the patient has just had a pulmonary embolism
    3. the capnometer tubing has been clogged with moisture
    4. there has been an increase in alveolar dead space

139. A mass spectrometer is a device that has been used to monitor gases and vapors from the airway of anesthetized patients. The primary analyzer is commonly used to monitor several rooms by sequentialing sampling gases from each room in sequence. This has the disadvantage of not providing continuous information from all rooms simultaneously. In spite of this disadvantage it has been used for over a decade because
    1. it is an inexpensive device
    2. it can be moved easily from room to room
    3. it quickly retrieves samples from multiple rooms
    4. it can measure all gases and vapors

140. Although mercury thermometers have been used for years to measure a patient's temperature, in the operating rooms we have relied upon thermistors and thermocouples because
    1. mercury thermometers are not sufficiently accurate
    2. mercury thermometers are much too expensive
    3. thermistors and thermocouples are more accurate
    4. mercury thermometers are brittle and pose a patient hazard

141. A recent article in the literature compares the effects of drug A and drug B on increasing cardiac output in patients in cardiogenic shock. In a prospective randomized blinded fashion, either drug is infused into a patient who meets the entrance criteria. After 20 patients have been enrolled in the study (10 in each group), the data are evaluated. A "T"-test resulted in a p value of greater than 0.05, and therefore, the drugs do not differ in their effect on cardiac output. What can be stated with respect to these results?
    1. drugs A and B have an equivalent effect on cardiac output with patients in cardiogenic shock
    2. drugs A and B do not have a significantly different effect on cardiac output in these patients
    3. nothing can be stated regarding these two drugs
    4. drugs A and B do have a different effect, but not in these patients

142. A trauma patient undergoing an emergency laparotomy is being resuscitated with warmed fluids and blood and is ventilated with a heated humidified circuit. In spite of these efforts the patient's temperature continues to fall. The anesthesiologist asks that the room temperature be raised by 5°F. In the next half hour the patient's temperature stabilizes and begins to rise. Why were the first two efforts ineffective in maintaining the patient's temperature while just raising the room temperature appeared to resolve the problem?
    1. blood warmers are usually unable to heat blood to 37°C
    2. most of the heat is lost to conduction, convection, and radiation, all of which are affected by room temperature
    3. humidifiers add too much cold water to the patient
    4. heating and humidifying the respiratory gases can save only 10% to 15% of the heat loss

143. A patient who is undergoing an exploratory laparotomy has a temperature of 35°C and falling, in spite of being ventilated with heated humidified gas and having been placed on a heating blanket maintained at 37°C. Which of the following mechanism(s) is (are) responsible for this problem?
   1. forced and natural convection
   2. latent heat of respiratory water vapor
   3. electromagnetic radiation
   4. conduction from the operating room into the table

Physics, Equipment, and Monitoring

Answers and Discussion

The authors have made every effort to thoroughly verify the answers to the questions that appear on the preceding pages. As in any text, however, some inaccuracies and ambiguities may occur. If in doubt, please consult the indicated reference. When no page number(s) are cited, the reference is to a journal article or to a refresher course lecture that should be read in its entirety.

The Editors

111. **(D)** Microshock is defined as a current below perceptible level, or lower than 1 mA. Macroshock refers to gross amounts of current, which can cause damage by tissue injury as well as by dysrhythmias. Microshock affects only those patients who have current paths of low resistance, such as open chest/fluid-filled catheters in which tiny currents can cause dysrhythmias. The division between microshock and macroshock is rather arbitrary. (**Ref. 7**, pp. 185–186)

112. **(D)** Electrocautery works by generating a very high frequency current (500,000 to 1 million Hz), which at high current density causes the cutting or coagulating of the "Bovie." The energy returns to the unit via a low-density return plate so that the energy

is dispersed and little heat is generated. This is why the "Bovie" can't coagulate a pool of blood (current density is too low to heat the blood) or can burn the patient if the return pad is improperly attached. Very high frequency current decreases the risk of fibrillation, which would be very high if 60 Hz current were to be used. (**Ref. 7,** pp. 198–202)

113. **(E)** X-rays are a powerful form of electromagnetic energy. As such they can remove electrons from orbits and ionize atoms. This energy can be quantified as activity (curies, $1 \text{ Ci} = 3.7 \times 10^{10}$ disintegrations per second), exposure (roentgen, $1 \text{ R} = 2.58 \times 10^{-4}$ C/kg of air), absorption (rad or grays, $1 \text{ rad} = 0.01$ Gray $= 0.01$ J/kg (energy into tissue), or biologic damage (rem = roentgen-equivalent-man). Backward-scattered radiation tends to be more intense than forward-scattered radiation. Exposure is proportional to the activity and inversely proportional to the square of the distance from the source. (**Ref. 7,** p. 179)

114. **(E)** Only flowmeter flows are affected. Proportioning systems work via either mechanical or pneumatic linkages to maintain an oxygen concentration of 25% or greater at the fresh gas outlet by altering the flowmeter flows. For this reason, they cannot detect proper gas supply from pipeline or cylinder or circuit leaks at any point in the system. Additionally, proportioning systems interface only with nitrous oxide and therefore cannot detect if a third gas (helium or nitrogen) is added in hypoxic quantities. (**Ref. 7,** pp. 645–647)

115. **(C)** Desflurane vapor pressure is very high, requiring a special vaporizer. It is otherwise very inert, does not degrade in soda lime, nor corrode metals. The MAC of desflurane is 6% and the vaporizer output is calibrated from 0% to 18% to allow for overpressure. (**Ref. 7,** p. 652)

116. **(B)** The oxygen flowmeter is last in line so that if a leak develops, oxygen will not be lost in greater proportion than the other gases. The oxygen flow control knob is fluted, larger, and projects out farther to distinguish it from knobs for other gases. Fail-safe valves prevent or reduce the flow of nitrous oxide as oxygen pressure decreases. Vaporizers include interlock systems to prevent more than one being active at any one time (avoids formation of

azeotropic mixtures and inadvertent overdoses). The vaporizers also have key indexing to prevent misfilling of the vaporizer. (**Ref. 7,** pp. 637–653)

117. **(B)** A suction bulb is required for the 1992 draft check-out. Both checks can detect vaporizer leaks, scavenging system, and CO_2 absorbent. The new draft requires that the following be present: ascending bellows ventilator, capnograph, pulse oximeter, oxygen analyzer, spirometer, and breathing system pressure monitor with both high- and low-pressure alarms. The suction bulb is required since some modern anesthesia machines have check valves that prevent leak detection via a simple positive pressure test. (**Ref. 36,** pp. 990–997)

118. **(D)** The volume in the tank is not proportional to the pressure, because nitrous oxide is not an ideal gas at room temperature. The pressure remains at the saturated vapor pressure (725 psi at room temperature) until all the liquid is evaporated, after which it rapidly declines. Blue is both the American and international standard color for nitrous oxide. (**Ref. 13,** pp. 3–8)

119. **(B)** Isotopes have the same number of protons and electrons, but differ in number of neutrons. They therefore have a different atomic mass but the same atomic number. Chemically, isotopes act identically (i.e., C_{14} is chemically indistinguishable from C_{12}). Many isotopes are radioactive, however, and emit various decay products or even change into different elements until they reach a stable atomic configuration. (**Ref. 33,** pp. 31–32)

120. **(A)** At a given pressure head, the flow through a tube is inversely proportionate to the length and directly proportional to the fourth power of the radius (Hagen–Poiseuille Law)

$$Q = \frac{\pi R^4}{8\mu L} \Delta P$$

Where Q = fluid flow rate, π = 3.14, R = radius, μ = viscosity of the fluid, L = length, and ΔP = pressure drop.

Thus, the shortest catheter with the largest diameter will permit the greatest flow. Given the choices, either A or D would be the greatest flow. Calculating as follows:

$$Q \propto \frac{R^4}{L}$$

(A) $\frac{1^4}{1.5} = 0.66$

(D) $\frac{(1.2)^4}{6} = \frac{2.07}{6} = 0.34$

Therefore A is the correct answer. (**Ref. 7,** p. 148)

121. (D) The volume of an E-cylinder is approximately 5 liters, and atmospheric pressure is approximately 15 PSIG (actually 14.7 PSIG). Therefore, the oxygen in the cylinder can be approximated by:

$$\frac{1000 \text{ PSIG}}{15 \text{ PSI/atmosphere}} = 66 \text{ atmosphere}$$

The volume will expand 66 times if it is reduced to atmospheric pressure. Consequently, the cylinder contains approximately 330 liters of oxygen.

$66 \times 5 = 330$ liters

At 2 liters per minute the oxygen would last approximately 165 minutes, or 2 hours and 45 minutes. (**Ref. 7,** pp. 152–153)

122. (E) Infrared absorption can measure only molecules that are asymmetric. Oxygen and nitrogen are diatomic molecules that are symmetric and therefore do not absorb infrared light. Raman scattering analyzers can analyze any molecule, for they measure a spectrum of emitted energy induced by excited bonds between the atoms. Therefore, to be detected by a Raman scattering device, a substance must have bonds and therefore at least two atoms. Mass spectrometers separate particles on the basis of charge to mass ratio and therefore do not require bonds and can measure single atoms as well as complex molecules. (**Ref. 32,** pp. 981–984)

123. **(C)** Use of bipolar cautery and physical monitoring are both important in patients with pacemakers. Electrical cautery can cause interference with the sensing of cardiac action potentials and cause inappropriate discharge or lack of discharge of the pacemaker. This interference is minimized by the use of bipolar cautery and/or placement of the return electrode away from the heart. A physical method of monitoring the pulse (a finger on the pulse) is to be recommended, since it is immune to electrical interference. (**Ref. 5,** p. 173)

124. **(C)** The two work in conjunction. Macroshock means that a current source must be applied to an electrically susceptible patient. Grounding would make the patient more electrically susceptible, whereas grounding the equipment would provide an alternate, low-resistance path and protect the patient. Nonconductive tubing can store a charge and create a spark (microshock or flame hazard). A faulty ground can be detected by the Line Isolation Monitor, and this should lead to the removal of a macroshock hazard. (**Ref. 7,** pp. 183–202)

125. **(B)** Scavenging does occur, and the driving gas is either 100% O_2 (for Ohmeda electronic ventilators) or a Venturi effect O_2 and air mixture (for Drager ventilators). Ascending bellows are felt to be safer because during a "disconnect" the ventilator bellows collapse. Scavenging does not occur during the inspiratory phase of positive pressure ventilation, leading to a risk of barotrauma if the oxygen flush is accidentally or intentionally activated during inspiration. (**Ref. 7,** pp. 660–669)

126. **(C)** Optical isolation protects both the patient and the machine. Prior to isolation, an ECG would have to be disconnected during defibrillation to prevent the amplifier from burning up during the high-power discharge. (**Ref. 33,** pp. 487–492)

127. **(A)** Ion-selective electrodes work by movement of ions across a selective membrane to establish an electrochemical signal, which is then amplified to produce a read-out. The solubility product constant determines the amount of material present before precipitation occurs. The Nernst equation determines the potential across a semipermeable membrane. (**Ref. 27,** pp. 617–619)

Answers and Discussion: 123–133 / 77

128. (B) Optimum mesh size was determined empirically as a balance between surface area and resistance to flow. The optimum volume must be greater than a tidal volume to allow for complete exchange of CO_2. Nonrebreathing circuits do not require CO_2 absorbers. (**Ref. 7,** pp. 653–658)

129. (E) Electrocautery can totally mask the ECG signal, whereas the 60 Hz current can be filtered. Since the ECG is a measurement of small electrical potentials, it can detect the myopotentials in the chest wall. Roller pumps used in cardiac surgery have been reported to alter the ECG as a function of the rate of pumping. (**Ref. 7,** pp. 771–775)

130. (A) Valves prevent expired gases from entering the inspiratory limb of the circle. If fresh gas flow entered between the expiratory valve and patient, expired gases would be forced to the patient. If the pop-off valve were between the patient and the inspiratory valve, fresh gas would exit the system rather than be delivered to the patient. If the CO_2 absorber is intact and functioning, the O_2 flows can be as low as the O_2 consumption without rebreathing CO_2. (**Ref. 7,** pp. 653–658)

131. (A) An E oxygen cylinder in the United States is color-coded green and contains 660 liters of gas at 1900 psi. White is the Canadian color. The volume of the cylinder can be calculated by the ideal gas law, PV = nRT, because oxygen is an ideal gas at these temperatures (and if one knew the number of moles of oxygen per liter at room temperature). (**Ref. 13,** pp. 3–8)

132. (A) A DC current produces a unidirectional voltage spike. (AC current alternates and is bidirectional.) Blocking the ECG electrodes may lead to the administration of an unnecessary, second shock. Because the ECG signal is on the order of millivolts, the large 300 Joule shock can damage the amplifiers if they are not protected. As with any energy discharge, skin burns are possible if the current density is high enough. (**Ref. 33,** pp. 487–492)

133. (A) The Bain circuit is a coaxial modification of the Mapleson D circuit. Because it consists of two tubes within each other, it is small in bulk and convenient for positioning patients. Flows should be greater than minute ventilation to prevent rebreathing.

This requirement makes the Bain circuit very expensive to operate and very wasteful of oxygen, nitrous oxide, and other inhalational anesthetic agents. All circuits should be scavenged to prevent contamination of the operating room environment with waste gases. (**Ref. 13,** pp. 103–108, 124)

134. (E) Beer's Law states that the light absorbed is proportional to (a) the concentration of the solute, (b) the path length of light, and (c) the absorbance coefficient of the solute. This is true for each of the solutes in solution, which absorb light at the wavelength of light being employed. (**Ref. 32,** pp. 981–982)

135. (D) A correlation coefficient determines only the degree of linear association. 1.0 is perfect positive linear association, and 0.0 is no linear association. To assess how the two relate numerically, you must know the slope and intercept. A correlation coefficient is not the best way to assess the numerical agreement between two methods of measurement. This is best assessed by measuring the bias (the mean difference between the two measurements) and the precision (the standard deviation of the differences). The bias represents the systematic error between the two methods of measurement, and the precision represents the random error. (**Ref. 32,** pp. 995–997)

136. (A) Amplification artifacts are common in fluid-filled transducer systems for measuring invasive blood pressure. The amplification of the systolic pressure increases as the primary frequency (pulse rate) approaches the natural resonance frequency of the system. The natural resonance frequency is determined by the volume of fluid contained in the system, the compliance of the system, and the friction associated with movement of fluid in the system. In the example above anything that increases the volume of liquid between the catheter tip and the transducer will increase the amplification artifact. Therefore, both increasing diameter of the arterial catheter and increasing length of the fluid-filled high-pressure tubing will increase the amplification artifact. As the pulse rate increases, the primary frequency approaches the natural resonance frequency; therefore, increasing pulse rate or tachycardia will also worsen the amplification artifact. Small bubbles inside the tubing will also increase the artifact by increasing the effective compliance of the tubing and also changing the friction within the tubing. (**Ref. 32,** pp. 960–962)

137. **(D)** Because a pulse oximeter uses two wave lengths of light, it can only estimate the proportion of oxyhemoglobin to reduced hemoglobin. The algorithm used in calibrating pulse oximeters is unable to account for the presence of carboxyhemoglobin. Since carboxyhemoglobin is red and absorbs red light to a similar degree as oxyhemoglobin, a pulse oximeter will read approximately the combined percentages of both. Therefore, the pulse oximeter is unable to determine the presence or absence of carboxyhemoglobin in the arterial blood. To determine the level of carboxyhemoglobin, an arterial sample must be sent for analysis on a laboratory cooximeter that uses multiple wavelengths of light to determine oxyhemoglobin, methemoglobin, reduced hemoglobin, and carboxyhemoglobin levels. (**Ref. 32,** pp. 986–987)

138. **(C)** In a healthy patient, the end expired CO_2 value of the alveolar plateau of the capnogram is usually within a few millimeters of mercury of the arterial CO_2 value. The difference between the arterial CO_2 and the end-expired value is determined by the proportion of well-perfused and ventilated alveoli to the nonperfused and ventilated alveoli (i.e., alveolar dead space). Nonperfused alveoli do not pick up CO_2, and therefore during expiration when the alveoli empty, their contents (alveolar dead space gas) dilutes the well-perfused alveolar gas ($\approx PaCO_2$), thereby lowering the end-expired CO_2 value. Alveolar dead space may increase due to a pulmonary embolism or a decrease in cardiac output or any hemodynamic or pulmonary change that would increase the ventilation–perfusion ratio. (**Ref. 8,** pp. 53–55)

139. **(D)** A mass spectrometer is an expensive device that is economically feasible only when multiplexed to several rooms. Because it analyzes ionized particles on the basis of charge to mass ratio, it is able to analyze all anesthetic vapors and respiratory gases as well as nitrogen, oxygen, and helium. None of the other currently available devices can measure all these components. (**Ref. 32,** pp. 974, 981–984)

140. **(D)** A mercury thermometer may break, thus posing a potential hazard of injury and mercury poisoning. Thermistors and thermocouples are inexpensive and flexible and may be placed in a variety of locations on the patient—for example, on the tip of a thermodilution pulmonary artery catheter or a urinary catheter. They also are incorporated into flexible esophageal stethoscopes. A mercury thermometer is a thermal expansion device and is based on the principle of thermal expansion to measure temperature, whereas a thermocouple relies on the Seebeck effect. (**Ref. 32,** pp. 974, 981–984)

141. **(C)** In this study, the null hypothesis was that there was a difference between these two drugs. This null hypothesis was disproven so that it can be stated that no significant difference can be found between the drugs. That does not mean, however, that the drugs are equivalent. A p value determines the probability of a type-1 error: What is the probability of there not being a difference when the data appear to show a difference? That is, a p-value of less than 0.05 means there is a 95% chance that there truly is a difference and only a 5% chance that there is no difference. To prove that the drugs are equivalent, you must rule out a type-2 error, that is, assuming that the drugs are equivalent when they are really not. For this the study would require a power analysis to determine the sample size required to prove that these two drugs are truly equivalent. Most frequently the sample size is chosen to prove this statement to a power of 80% (i.e., there is an 80% chance that the drugs are equivalent and only a 20% chance that they are not). Statements regarding equivalency of the two drugs, therefore, can be made only if a power analysis has been performed. (**Ref. 2,** pp. 1336–1338)

142. **(B)** Patients lose heat by four mechanisms: conduction, convection (forced and natural), radiation, and latent heat of vaporization. To lose heat by conduction, the patient must be in contact with a surface at a lower temperature. To lose heat by latent heat of vaporization, a liquid must vaporize. Heat loss caused by forced and natural convection requires a fluid contact (air) that is either blown across the patient or moved by natural currents. This patient is predominantly losing heat because of convection and radiation from the exposed portions of the patient to the room. The patient should not be losing any heat by conduction into the

table if it is maintained at the same temperature as the body, or above it. There also should be no heat loss as a result of respiratory water vaporization if the patient is breathing 100% humidified gas at body temperature. (**Ref. 7,** pp. 158–162)

143. (C) An anesthetized patient will lose heat immediately upon entering a cold room by the mechanisms of conduction, convection, and radiation. A patient with normal temperature and metabolism will generate approximately 100 watts, of which only 10% to 15% are due to the latent heat of vaporization of respiratory water. All the mechanisms of heat loss are dramatically affected by the surrounding temperature. If the room were 37°C, the patient could not lose any heat except for latent heat of vaporization, and the room may increase in temperature due to the heat produced by the patient's metabolism. New efficient blood and fluid warmers can heat blood to 37°, but that maintains only the patient's temperature and cannot add significantly to it. Having the patient breathe heated humidified gases has similar effects. (**Ref. 7,** pp. 158–162)

6

Anesthesia for General Surgery

DIRECTIONS (Questions 144–173): For each of the questions or incomplete answers below, **one** or **more** of the answers or completions are correct. Select
- **A.** if only 1, 2, and 3 are correct
- **B.** if only 1 and 3 are correct
- **C.** if only 2 and 4 are correct
- **D.** if only 4 is correct
- **E.** if all are correct

144. The patients who are most likely to experience acid reflux in the perioperative period are patients with a history of
    1. familial dysautonomia
    2. dermatomyositis
    3. alcoholism
    4. Down syndrome

145. The anesthetic risks in emergency surgery for acute peptic ulcer disease include
    1. gastric reflux and aspiration
    2. difficult reversal of neuromuscular blockers

3. blood pressure sensitive to anesthetic agents
4. slow awakening from general anesthesia

146. Preventive measures against acid reflux and aspiration during the perioperative period may include
    1. having the patient take aluminum or magnesium antacid tablets one hour preoperatively
    2. the administration of oral Bicitra 90 minutes preoperatively
    3. the intravenous injection of cimetidine with induction
    4. delaying extubation until the patient is awake

147. In patients undergoing insulinoma removal
    1. continuous monitoring of plasma glucose is essential
    2. maintenance of moderate hypoglycemia is advisable
    3. plasma glucose monitoring is not necessary
    4. intermittent plasma glucose sampling is adequate to protect patients from hypoglycemia

148. Biliary cirrhosis is characterized by
    1. pathology primarily in the periportal areas
    2. porto-systemic shunting
    3. increased cardiac output
    4. decreased total body water

149. In the patient requiring surgery who has concomitant liver disease, the following would be good indicators of hepatic function:
    1. sensitivity to catecholamines
    2. increased prothrombin time
    3. reduced drug requirements
    4. reduced serum proteins

150. Medications to be used with caution, if at all, in endoscopic cholecystectomy surgery include
    1. atropine
    2. morphine
    3. glucagon
    4. meperidine

84 / 6: Anesthesia for General Surgery

151. A 60-kg patient, after three hours of abdominal surgery under N_2O, O_2 isoflurane anesthesia with pancuronium (10 mg total dose) is having her abdominal muscle fascia closed. There are one weak and two weaker twitches on ulnar nerve stimulation by train-of-four. The surgeon is having difficulty closing. At this point, the most appropriate maneuver to facilitate closure would be to
    1. administer 100 mg IV succinylcholine
    2. increase the isoflurane concentration
    3. administer 2.0 mg IV pancuronium
    4. administer 0.5 mg IV pancuronium

152. A patient is given a spinal anesthetic for a herniorrhaphy. The level to pin prick is T_6. Causes for nausea and vomiting in this case might be
    1. vagal afferent stimulation from testicular traction
    2. central stimulation from vasopressor used to treat hypotension
    3. cerebral ischaemia from hypotension
    4. hyperperistalsis from sympathetic blockade

153. Which of the following makes it more likely that the patient will regurgitate perioperatively?
    1. esophageal hiatus hernia
    2. Zenker's diverticulum
    3. postviral gastroparesis
    4. nasogastric tube

154. In anesthetizing a patient with hepatic failure, which of the following drugs would have a slower onset of action?
    1. pancuronium
    2. atracurium
    3. vecuronium
    4. metocurine

155. In awakening an intubated patient, who may have liquid or particulate gastric contents, what precautions should be taken?
    1. liquid antacid instillation by nasogastric tube
    2. aspiration of stomach contents prior to emergence
    3. determination of no fade-in train-of-four nerve stimulation
    4. confirmation of ability to swallow on command

156. During laparoscopic cholecystectomy
   1. the blood pressure and pulse are usually stable
   2. the peak inspiratory pressures may rise
   3. low-flow system use is inadvisable
   4. CO_2 absorber granule consumption may increase

157. Which signs indicate the development of a carbon dioxide embolus?
   1. a sudden fall in expired CO_2 on the capnogram
   2. a mill-wheel murmur
   3. a fall in arterial oxygen saturation
   4. hypotension and tachycardia

158. Venous air embolism may be treated by
   1. applying positive end expiratory pressure
   2. maintaining reverse Trendelenburg position
   3. infusing a 300 mL IV crystalloid bolus
   4. shutting off N_2O and flushing the breathing circuit with oxygen

159. Complications of laparoscopic surgery may include
   1. significant blood loss
   2. delayed recovery from neuromuscular blockade
   3. venous gas embolism
   4. increased gastroesophageal competence

160. The serious postoperative complications of pancreatoduodenectomy include
   1. coagulopathy
   2. hemorrhage
   3. multiple organ system failure
   4. pulmonary failure

161. The severity of pulmonary insult from aspiration is a function of
   1. hypoxia
   2. pH and volume
   3. hypercarbia
   4. the presence or absence of particulate matter

86 / 6: Anesthesia for General Surgery

162. Which of the following would make it difficult for a patient to breathe adequately following a laparotomy?
1. supine position
2. general anesthesia
3. Trendelenburg position
4. abdominal pain

163. Temperature regulation in an aged patient may be compromised by
1. decreased non-shivering thermogenesis
2. sweat gland atrophy
3. slowing lipolysis rates with aging
4. increased noradrenergic receptor sensitivity

164. General anesthesia for an intra-abdominal procedure may produce heat loss as a result of
1. lowering the thermostatic set point
2. large surface area prep
3. peripheral arteriolar vasodilatation
4. semiclosed breathing system

165. A patient had blunt trauma to the abdomen. Peritoneal lavage reveals some blood. The presence of blood suggests
1. splenic rupture
2. retroperitoneal bleeding
3. hepatic laceration
4. bowel perforation

166. What implications does a positive peritoneal lavage for blood hold for the anesthesiologist?
1. the intravascular volume status should be assessed
3. a prophylactic antibiotic should be administered
2. blood should be ordered
4. the Trendelenburg position should be avoided

167. In an obese patient, the Trendelenburg position is requested by the surgeon for better abdominal access. The anesthesiologist should expect that
1. the functional residual capacity will not change
2. the residual volume will decrease

3. the inspiratory reserve capacity will not be reduced
4. the closing capacity will not change

168. With respect to the carcinoid syndrome
    1. 65% of the patients with carcinoid tumors have carcinoid syndrome
    2. the appearance of symptoms is related to metastasis
    3. bronchospasm is rare, and mild if it does appear
    4. somatostatin is effective in preventing or treating symptoms intraoperatively

169. In a patient with a duodenal obstruction
    1. serum potassium will be low
    2. potassium is lost in the gastric fluid
    3. hypochloremic alkalosis develops
    4. potassium is excreted by the kidney

170. In the presence of small bowel obstruction
    1. use of a jejunal suction tube will prevent regurgitation
    2. bowel dilatation may result in fluid loss into the bowel wall and into the peritoneal cavity
    3. use of an H_1 blocker is indicated
    4. contents proximal to the obstruction include increased secretions

171. Gastric suction in a patient with small bowel obstruction may lead to
    1. decreased blood volume
    2. total body potassium will drop
    3. metabolic acidosis will develop
    4. hypochloremia will develop

172. In the obese patient
    1. oxygen consumption is increased
    2. basal metabolic rate is increased
    3. carbon dioxide production is increased
    4. chest–lung compliance is reduced

173. Difficulties that may be encountered in establishing and maintaining an airway in an obese patient are
1. limited neck extension
2. the larynx may be high and anterior
3. limited neck flexion
4. limited mouth opening

Anesthesia for General Surgery

Answers and Discussion

The authors have made every effort to thoroughly verify the answers to the questions that appear on the preceding pages. As in any text, however, some inaccuracies and ambiguities may occur. If in doubt, please consult the indicated reference. When no page number(s) are cited, the reference is to a journal article or to a refresher course lecture that should be read in its entirety.

The Editors

144. (A) Any condition that may compromise neural or mechanical control of the esophagus may render the patient more likely to experience acid reflux. Besides the answers given, neurologic illnesses, gastric outlet obstruction, and other collagen vascular disorders such as polymyositis and scleroderma may have reflux as part of their clinical picture. Down syndrome is not one of these. (**Ref. 36,** p. 1969)

145. (B) The blood volume status of these patients, and therefore their sensitivity to anesthetic agents, can change rapidly. The stomach and the small and large bowels may contain significant amounts of blood. The patient must be considered to have a full stomach with acid contents. There is no consistent biochemical,

90 / 6: Anesthesia for General Surgery

physiologic, or pharmacologic change that will alter the patient's response to muscle relaxants or to general anesthetic agents. (**Ref. 36,** p. 1973)

146. **(D)** Particulate antacids are capable of being as destructive to the lungs as acid reflux. Soluble antacids have lost much of their effectiveness by one and a half hours. Cimetidine will not affect gastric acidity at the time of its injection. Delaying extubation improves the patient's ability to deal with any acid reflux. Conformational changes in the patient's larynx may result from the intubation, and temporarily may render glottic closure incomplete. Having the muscle relaxant fully reversed and the patient awake and oriented at the time of extubation is optimal. (**Ref. 36,** p. 1982)

147. **(D)** Intermittent sampling of plasma glucose is adequate. Maintaining moderate hypoglycemia affords no reserve in the event of subsequent boluses of insulin released by surgical manipulation of the insulinoma, whereas maintaining a moderate hyperglycemia does. Transient hyperglycemia is not injurious, whereas a period of hypoglycemia may be injurious or even disastrous. Following removal of the tumor, rebound hyperglycemia may occur, but it is not difficult to deal with. (**Ref. 26,** pp. 281–282)

148. **(A)** Periportal pathology results in portal hypertension and shunting of the venous blood away from the portal circulation. There is a relative increase in the contribution of the hepatic artery, as a consequence of this shunting. This renders the liver more vulnerable to systemic arterial hypoxia and hypotension. Characteristic of chronic liver disease is a high-output state with flushed extremities. A vasodilator substance is either produced by, or is not inactivated by the damaged liver. There is, however, reduced renal plasma flow leading to hepatorenal failure in the later stages of chronic liver disease. Water retention, hyponatremia, azotemia, and oliguria are consequences of this reduced renal plasma flow. (**Ref. 26,** p. 517)

149. **(C)** The liver produces most of the blood procoagulant and inhibitor factors. It also produces most of the serum proteins. Because of shunting, vasodilator substance levels may be increased, rendering the patient relatively insensitive to catecholamine-like

drugs. Reduced drug requirements are not a sensitive indicator of hepatic function. Removal of half the liver mass results in only transient changes in function. Given the usual patient-to-patient variation in drug sensitivity, liver function changes should be evident in specific function studies before they become apparent in changed drug requirements. (**Ref. 36,** pp. 318, 1999)

150. **(C)** Nitroglycerin, atropine, and glucagon may be used to reverse opiate-related biliary spasm. Therapeutic doses of the opioids can cause a marked rise in biliary tract pressure. The usual analgesic dose of morphine can produce a marked rise in common bile duct pressure that can last two or more hours. The commonly used anesthetic opiates, fentanyl and alfentanyl, and probably also sufentanyl, also raise the common bile duct pressure. Opiate antagonists such as naloxone can antagonize this opiate-related increase in biliary tract pressure, but this effect may be at the expense of the analgesia the opiates may be providing. Nitroglycerin, 0.6 mg sublingually, decreases the elevated intrabiliary pressure. Atropine may be partially effective. Glucagon, 1–3 mg IV will reverse biliary spasm resulting from opiate administration. (**Ref. 36,** p. 1984)

151. **(D)** Administering a paralyzing dose of succinylcholine to a patient who has been given a nondepolarizing relaxant during the same anesthetic may prolong the nondepolarizing block. Additionally, the onset of its effect under these circumstances would not be significantly faster than the administration of an appropriate dose of the nondepolarizer previously used. If a dose of 10 mg pancuronium has been adequate to relax this patient for a 3-hour procedure, 0.5 mg should be sufficient to deepen her relaxation significantly and quickly. Two mg would be excessive and might make the patient difficult to reverse at the end of the procedure. Turning off the N_2O, especially at low flows, it would take a long time to flush out the N_2O from the bowel. N_2O is the most insoluble of the inhaled anesthetics, so its absorption through a limited surface area of bowel mucosa and subsequent elimination through the lungs would be slow. Increasing the isoflurane concentration would increase relaxation too slowly and might cause hypotension. Increasing isoflurane concentration moderately would synergize with pancuronium administration. (**Ref. 36,** p. 1983)

152. **(E)** Parasympathetic afferent stimulation from testicular traction may not be blocked by spinal anesthesia adequate for motor and sensory blockade of the operative area. Noncatecholamine vasopressors may have central stimulating properties (ephedrine). An early symptom of cerebral ischaemia in an awake patient may be nausea, resulting from cerebral hypoxia. Sympathetic blockade of the abdominal sympathetic efferent rami may allow hyperperistalsis from unopposed vagal tone. (**Ref. 36,** p. 2054, **41,** pp. 222, 263, 619–620)

153. **(A)** A hiatus hernia produces a defect in esophageal propulsion that can allow passive regurgitation of stomach contents. A Zenker's diverticulum may sequester food contents in the hypopharynx, which could empty from the diverticulum while the patient is asleep or awake. Postviral gastroparesis may cause delayed gastric emptying, allowing the accumulation of stomach contents. A nasogastric tube, properly used, should reduce at least some liquid and gas accumulation in the stomach and reduce the likelihood of regurgitation. (**Ref. 36,** p. 1969)

154. **(E)** Because of the increased volume of distribution expected in these patients, there may be both a slower onset of action and a larger dose requirement for a given level of relaxation when using these relaxants. The increased volume into which the dose is injected results in a lower initial plasma concentration for any drug. Once adequate relaxation is established, the metabolism of only atracurium is undiminished. This property could be advantageous if the procedure is short. (**Ref. 36,** p. 2003)

155. **(C)** Aspiration will minimize the volume and the pressure of the stomach contents, decreasing the likelihood of clinically significant regurgitation. The patient's ability to follow commands, and particularly to swallow, indicates the ability to clear regurgitated stomach contents. There is no guarantee that instilled liquid antacid will mix adequately with stomach contents to neutralize all acid. The determination of "no fade" on train-of-four stimulation confirms only that approximately 30% of receptor sites are available for occupation by acetylcholine from motor nerve endings. That percentage represents an inadequate receptor site reserve for a patient who may experience repeated vomiting and/or coughing. (**Ref. 36,** p. 1982)

Answers and Discussion: 152–159 / 93

156. **(C)** The peak inspiratory pressures required for adequate ventilation may rise because of increased abdominal pressure against the diaphragm. Although CO_2 production is not increased, significant amounts of CO_2 are absorbed into the blood from the peritoneal cavity. This CO_2 requires removal through the lungs. Blood pressure and pulse may be unstable because of the damming back of venous return by increased intraabdominal pressure and also because of the restriction of return resulting from the head-up position. Use of a low-flow system is quite acceptable, but CO_2 absorber granule exhaustion will be significantly greater in these cases. (**Ref. 36,** pp. 1974, 2130)

157. **(E)** These are both the classic and also the newer signs of venous gas embolism. Even though additional CO_2 is being added to the blood, the pulmonary gas embolus is reducing perfusion of well-ventilated lungs. The capnogram shows a sudden drop in CO_2 output, since a reduced amount of CO_2 is mixed with the usual amount of gas ventilating the alveoli. Oxygen desaturation also results from this ventilation/perfusion mismatch. The millwheel murmur may result from the foaming of blood in the right ventricle and in the pulmonary outflow tract. Systemic hypotension and tachycardia result from the inadequate cardiac output caused by the gas embolus obstruction which reduces left ventricular preload. (**Ref. 36,** p. 2132)

158. **(D)** N_2O in the blood will diffuse into any air, CO_2 or other gas-filled space and will significantly increase the size of the space or the pressure within it. The N_2O must be removed from the blood as quickly as possible. PEEP is not useful in reducing the effect of the embolus. It synergizes with the embolus in reducing cardiac output. Nor is augmenting intravascular volume useful. There should be abundant preload available behind the embolus. Maintaining reverse Trendelenburg tends to promote embolization of the pulmonary outflow tract and to aggravate ventilation/perfusion mismatch and systemic hypotension from reduced left ventricular preload. (**Ref. 36,** p. 2132)

159. **(B)** The Verres needle or the trochar may lacerate a major artery or vein. CO_2 is administered under pressures greater than venous pressure, with the potential of introducing significant amounts of

CO_2 into the abdominal venous circulation. Anesthesia for laparoscopy does not involve an unusual risk for prolonged neuromuscular blockade. The increased pressure differential between stomach and thorax may promote gastroesophageal reflux. (**Ref. 36,** p. 1974)

160. (**E**) All those listed are possible complications of this procedure. This procedure is long in duration and extensive in area. It is traumatic to intraabdominal and retroperitoneal organs and to large surfaces of the parietal peritoneum. The anesthesiologist should be prepared to use invasive monitoring techniques and to monitor cardiac, pulmonary, and renal function very closely. There is potential for significant blood loss and for coagulopathy intraoperatively, and for hepatic, renal, pulmonary, and cardiovascular failure postoperatively. Optimization of the patient's condition preoperatively and conscientious attention to promoting optimal function intraoperatively will minimize the incidence of organ failure postoperatively. (**Ref. 36,** p. 1976)

161. (**C**) If a larger volume is aspirated and particularly if the aspirated volume exceeds 25 ml, it is more likely that the acid aspirate will reach enough alveoli to compromise pulmonary function. An aspirate having a pH of 2.5 or less is much more likely to produce pulmonary damage. Hypoxia and hypercarbia may be indications of the severity of the pulmonary injury but are not determinants of it. (**Ref. 36,** p. 1982)

162. (**E**) The supine position will reduce the FRC of a normal adult by 0.5 to 1.0 L. General anesthesia itself will reduce FRC by 15% to 20%. The Trendelenburg position, if it were used postoperatively for some reason, would also worsen ventilation/perfusion further by increasing the volume of lung in which pulmonary venous pressure exceeds alveolar pressure. It would also necessitate increased work of breathing, requiring the weight of the abdominal contents to be raised with each breath. The added hydrostatic pressure distends the pulmonary vessels, leaving less room for alveolar ventilation. Abdominal pain can prevent the patient from breathing efficiently with deep breaths. The patient limits respiratory excursions to minimize wound distortion (splinting). (**Ref. 36,** p. 1984)

163. (A) Nonshivering thermogenesis is largely mediated by norepinephrine. In the aged, there is both an increased serum level of norepinephrine and a decreased noradrenergic receptor sensitivity. This renders added norepinephrine less effective in accomplishing thermoregulation. Sweat gland atrophy limits the ability of the aged patient to compensate for excessive temperature levels. Stress-induced and insulin-induced lipolysis are reduced in the aged, limiting energy for heat production from lipolysis. (**Ref. 26,** p. 220)

164. (E) General anesthetics disrupt the preoptic and hypothalamic nuclear coordination of thermoregulation. They also result in generalized vasodilatation, which makes more heat available at the surface, to be lost through evaporation during the extensive skin preparation. A semiclosed breathing system exhausts a large percentage of the exhaled gases, which carry most of their heat with them. In a closed system, heat from exhaled gases tends to be preserved. (**Ref. 26,** p. 220)

165. (B) The most common injuries shown by a heme-positive peritoneal lavage are splenic rupture and hepatic laceration. These are the two most rigid intraperitoneal organs, and both are well perfused. This renders them the most likely organs to show damage by loss of blood into the peritoneal cavity. Lavage in the presence of bowel perforation would result in a wash contaminated with feces. Bowel has a lower mass for a given area, and it is relatively free to yield to a traumatic blow without sustaining significant damage. Retroperitoneal bleeding may be detectable by means of lavage only if the trauma has also lacerated the parietal peritoneum. Retroperitoneal bleeding may be extensive without there being blood in the peritoneal lavage. (**Ref. 7,** pp. 1420–1421)

166. (B) The positive lavage indicates bleeding but does not indicate the amount. Therefore, intravascular volume status should be assessed, and blood should be ordered. Other clinical signs and symptoms will allow estimation of the quantity of blood loss. If there is no indication of fecal contamination, there is no reason, based on lavage results, to use antibiotic prophylaxis. Splenic or hepatic bleeding is the most likely cause of a positive tap, depending on the area of the trauma. It would be pointless to attempt to avoid getting blood under the diaphragm by avoiding the Trendelenburg position. (**Ref. 7,** p. 1420)

167. **(C)** With greater extrinsic pressure on the thorax from the added weight on the diaphragm in the supine position, the expiratory reserve volume and the functional residual capacity diminish in the obese person. Closing capacity (CC) is low in the inspiratory reserve volume. The Trendelenburg position in the obese worsens matters. Now both inspiratory reserve volume (IRV) and residual volume are reduced in addition, and CC may be found high in the IRV. Closing capacity is the point in the vital capacity tracing at which some respiratory units no longer contribute to expiratory flow. CC does not change with Trendelenburg position, so with increasing obesity, CC takes up more and more of the IRV of the patient. (**Ref. 7,** pp. 1169–1170)

168. **(C)** Symptoms of the carcinoid syndrome usually appear only after metastasis has taken place, since most primary tumors are located along the GI tract, and their hormones are inactivated as they pass through the liver. Once there are liver or other distant metastases, the tumor can secrete directly into the systemic circulation and cause symptoms. Somatostatin or ketanserin, antiserotonin drugs, are effective in the prophylaxis of intraoperative response. Only about 35% of patients with both tumors and metastases will have the symptoms of the syndrome. Bronchospasm occurs frequently enough and is severe enough that the use of prophylactic H_1 and H_2 blockers is advised. (**Ref. 7,** pp. 1180–1181)

169. **(E)** In a patient with duodenal obstruction, hydrochloric acid is vomited or suctioned from the stomach. The acid produced in the stomach and removed by this means leaves behind a complementary alkalinity in the blood. Potassium is excreted by the kidneys in response to the alkalosis to get rid of base. The alkalosis is hypochloremic because of the loss of chloride as hydrochloric acid. Some potassium is also lost in the vomitus or suction. (**Ref. 7,** p. 1179)

170. **(C)** Bowel wall edema can result from compromise to the venous circulation of the bowel by mechanical means, such as hernia or volvulus, or can result from bowel wall dilatation by intrin-

sic pressure or from other bowel disease. Bowel dilatation behind an obstruction may progress to necrosis and perforation. The contents behind the obstruction would include all the upstream bowel contents as well as secretions. Jejunal suction cannot be depended upon to prevent regurgitation of the bowel contents. An H_2 blocker would not affect the pH of the bowel contents, which could be nearly neutral in pH or even alkaline. (**Ref. 7,** p. 1179)

171. **(E)** The body will attempt to mobilize extracellular fluid to make up for the volume lost to suction. This mobilization will not ultimately keep up with loss. The blood volume will drop and the hematocrit will rise. The kidneys, in attempting to preserve intravascular volume, will not be able to excrete sufficient hydrogen ions to preserve homeostasis, and acidosis will ensue. Hypochloremia will result from losses to suction of gastric secretions. (**Ref. 7,** p. 1179)

172. **(B)** Since the basal metabolic rate is related to body surface area, it is not elevated, unlike oxygen consumption and CO_2 production, which increase when the tissue mass increases. Lung compliance remains relatively normal, and the chest wall compliance decreases by the fat mass on and in the thoracic wall. (**Ref. 7,** p. 1169)

173. **(E)** Neck flexion may be limited by thoracic wall fat, breast fat, or chin fat. Extension may be limited by low cervical or upper thoracic fat pads. The laryngeal aperture may be high and anterior. Mouth opening may be restricted by submental fat. An attempt to visualize the larynx is advisable before anesthetizing a patient. It may become apparent that an awake intubation is required. If fiberoptic equipment is available, it should be used electively in potentially difficult intubations. There is no justification for taking chances with the patient's life as long as a safe and relatively certain technique is available to secure the airway. (**Ref. 7,** p. 1171)

7
Anesthesia for Orthopedic Surgery

DIRECTIONS (Questions 174–200): For each of the questions or incomplete answers below, **one** or **more** of the answers or completions are correct. Select

    A. if only 1, 2, and 3 are correct
    B. if only 1 and 3 are correct
    C. if only 2 and 4 are correct
    D. if only 4 is correct
    E. if all are correct

---

174. During total hip replacement, hypotension may often be explained by
    1. fat embolism during packing of cement into the femoral shaft
    2. vasodilation from uptake of methylmethacrylate monomer
    3. blood loss
    4. parasympathetic outpouring from the hip joint capsule leading to vagally mediated bradycardia

175. A patient is to undergo lumbar laminectomy in the prone position. Precautions must include
  1. avoiding compression of the femoral nerve by overly long chest rolls, which can lead to meralgia paresthetica
  2. checking male genitalia to see that they are not distorted, compressed, or under traction by the urinary catheter
  3. turning the patient with arms extended overhead so as not to lose intravascular catheters
  4. supporting the head in the midline by a padded face rest or a three-prong skull clamp to prevent eye injury or blindness

176. The landmarks for a median nerve block at the elbow include the
  1. brachial artery
  2. medial epicondyle
  3. lateral epicondyle
  4. radial artery

177. The landmarks for a radial nerve block at the wrist are the
  1. tendon of the flexor carpi radialis
  2. radial artery
  3. tendon of the palmaris longus
  4. styloid process of the ulna

178. Advanced kyphoscoliosis may lead to which of the following?
  1. polycythemia
  2. right ventricular enlargement
  3. decreased tidal volume
  4. obstructive lung disease

179. Osteoarthritis
  1. commonly affects the hips, knees, hands, feet, and spine
  2. can cause Heberden's and Bouchard's nodes
  3. can be associated with a history of steroidal and nonsteroidal medication
  4. systemic manifestations are not uncommon

180. Rheumatoid arthritis
1. most commonly affects the hands, feet, wrists, and knees
2. affects about 10% of the population in the U.S., is more common in males, and is associated with the HLA B27 histocompatibility antigen
3. causes cervical spine fusion, limiting range of neck motion
4. can cause even asymptomatic patients to require surgical neck stabilization

181. Airway problems associated with rheumatoid arthritis include
1. temporomandibular joint erosion, leading to decreased mouth opening
2. anterior atlanto-axial subluxation in approximately 2% of patients
3. cricoarytenoid arthritis, leading to narrowing of the larynx
4. frequent and more dangerous anterior atlanto-axial subluxation

182. The extraarticular manifestations of rheumatoid arthritis include
1. pericarditis
2. macrocytic anemia
3. Caplan's syndrome
4. thrombocytopenia

183. Ankylosing spondylitis
1. affects approximately 1.6% of the population and is more severe in males
2. cardiac involvement is found in >3.5% of patients with a >15-year history
3. cervical spine films in flexion and extension should be obtained preoperatively
4. unlike in rheumatoid arthritis, the temporomandibular and cricoarytenoid joints are not affected

184. Which of the following statement(s) regarding anesthesia for total hip arthroplasty is (are) correct?
1. regional anesthesia can decrease blood loss by 30% to 50%
2. spontaneous respiration contributes to decreased venous bleeding

3. mean arterial pressure, pulmonary artery pressure, and peripheral venous pressure are all decreased during epidural anesthesia
4. during epidural anesthesia blood flow is redistributed to the upper limbs

185. Regarding hip surgery
    1. the incidence of deep vein thrombosis (DVT) following total hip arthroplasty (THA) is approximately 10%
    2. the incidence of pulmonary embolism (PE) following THA is approximately 2% to 3%
    3. regional anesthesia does not significantly reduce the incidence of DVT and PE
    4. hypotensive general anesthesia can reduce blood loss to an extent similar to that of regional anesthesia

186. Regional anesthesia may affect the risk of thromboembolism in which of the following ways?
    1. local anesthetics may reduce the adhesion of leukocytes to blood vessel walls
    2. the resting levels of plasminogen are increased
    3. increased blood flow occurs in the lower extremities
    4. it causes thrombocytosis

187. The complication(s) of total hip replacement include
    1. intraoperative hypotension and cardiopulmonary collapse during cementing of the femoral prosthesis
    2. methylmethacrylate monomer absorption into the bloodstream may cause systemic hypertension and myocardial infarction
    3. bone fragments, air, clots, and methylmethacrylate can be forced into open venous sinuses, causing thromboplastin release and platelet-fibrin aggregation in the pulmonary circulation
    4. decreases in PaO_2 at the time of femoral prosthesis placement is mostly likely related to profound vasodilation

188. Regarding sites of positional injury in orthopedic surgery
1. pressure at the elbow or traction of C_8–T_1 dermatomes over the first rib is not uncommon and leads to numbness of the ring and fifth fingers
2. pressure around the medial malleolus results in foot drop
3. pressure over the anterior iliac crest in the lateral or prone position or over the lateral thigh results in numbness of the lateral aspect of the thigh
4. pressure behind the upper arm results in numbness over the palm of the hand

189. In fractures of large bones
1. lung dysfunction is clinically significant after most fractures of long bones
2. fat embolism syndrome (FES) occurs in isolated long-bone fractures in approximately 3% to 4% of cases
3. mortality due to FES is approximately 50%
4. the incidence of FES increases with fractures of the pelvis

190. The criteria for the diagnosis of the fat embolism syndrome (FES) include(s) the following:
1. central nervous system depression disproportionate to the level of hypoxia
2. thrombocytopenia, increased erythrocyte sedimentation rate, increased fibrin degradation products, and a fall in hematocrit
3. retinal fat globules
4. reduced levels of free fatty acids, serum triglycerides, and serum lipase activity

191. Which of the following is (are) true concerning the anesthetic techniques used for hip surgery?
1. long-term survival rates have shown that regional anesthesia causes less mortality than general anesthesia
2. studies have shown a decreased mortality with spinal anesthesia when compared to general anesthesia from 2 to 4 weeks after the procedure
3. postoperative hypoxemia is similar after regional and general anesthesia
4. by two months there is no difference in mortality rates between spinal and general anesthesia

192. In scoliosis
1. approximately 75% to 90% of cases are idiopathic (genetic)
2. 70% to 85% of adolescent scoliotics are female
3. it may be a complicating factor in poliomyelitis, syringomyelia, and muscular dystrophy
4. patients with curvatures of more than 60° often have a respiratory pattern of obstructive pulmonary disease

193. In patients with severe scoliosis
1. vital capacity, total lung capacity, and functional residual capacity are all reduced
2. ventilation–perfusion mismatch is not usually a significant problem
3. chronic hypoxia may lead to pulmonary hypertension, cor pulmonale, and death
4. hypercapnia is an early sign of disease

194. In patients undergoing surgical repair of severe scoliosis
1. a vital capacity of <75% of predicted value often indicates a need for postoperative ventilation
2. there may be an altered response to CO_2 and an increased susceptibility to respiratory depression
3. a loud first heart sound is not uncommonly heard on auscultation
4. a preoperative ECG may show signs of right atrial dilation and right ventricular hypertrophy

195. What methods may be used to minimize homologous blood transfusion during scoliosis surgery?
1. hypotensive anesthesia
2. hemodilution
3. use of autologous blood donation
4. intraoperative red cell salvage and autotransfusion using the cell saver

196. Considering the tests of spinal cord function during scoliosis surgery
1. the wake-up test gives no false negatives but tests the anterior spinal cord (motor) function only
2. disadvantages of the wake-up test include inadvertent extubation, air embolism, and dislodgment of orthopedic hardware
3. the use of a nitrous oxide–narcotic–shorter-acting muscle relaxant anesthetic technique facilitates the wake-up test
4. tests of spinal cord function during surgery are usually unnecessary in adolescent scoliotic patients

197. Pneumatic arterial tourniquets
1. are used during surgery to decrease blood loss and to provide a relatively bloodless operative field
2. may cause an increase in blood pressure of 30% on inflation
3. lower limb exsanguination may transfuse up to 500 mL to the central circulation
4. deflation of a tourniquet can cause an acute increase in systemic vascular resistance (SVR)

198. Regarding pneumatic tourniquets used during surgery
1. tourniquet pressure on the lower limb should be higher than that on the upper limb due to the larger mass of the lower limb and the fact that femoral systolic pressure is higher than brachial systolic pressure
2. after two hours of tourniquet time there is mitochondrial swelling, myelin degeneration, and z-line lysis
3. tourniquet inflation pressure on the upper limb should be at least 50 mm Hg above systolic pressure
4. tourniquets must be deflated after a maximum of 4 hours

199. Changes seen with release of an arterial tourniquet include
1. PaO_2 may decrease by 20 to 30 mm Hg
2. PaO_2 and $PaCO_2$ may increase by 50 mm Hg
3. serum potassium may increase by >0.5 mEq/L
4. after one hour of leg ischemia time, the cooled limb will lower body temperature approximately 2.0°C

200. Complication(s) of arterial tourniquet use include
1. damage to blood vessels, skeletal muscle and peripheral nerves
2. nerve damage is thought to be primarily due to ischemia
3. nerve damage can be caused by improper tourniquet size, poor padding of the extremities, and high inflation pressure
4. tourniquet pain is an acute pain that usually occurs after 20 to 25 minutes of ischemia

Anesthesia for Orthopedic Surgery

Answers and Discussion

The authors have made every effort to thoroughly verify the answers to the questions that appear on the preceding pages. As in any text, however, some inaccuracies and ambiguities may occur. If in doubt, please consult the indicated reference. When no page number(s) are cited, the reference is to a journal article or to a refresher course lecture that should be read in its entirety.

The Editors

174. (A) Sudden hypotension and even cardiovascular collapse and death have resulted from overly vigorous packing of methylmethacrylate cement. The hypotension may be due to the vasodilatory effect of the cement monomers escaping into the blood stream, to emboli forced into the circulation as the prosthesis is inserted into a reamed and curetted medullary bone, to the effects of heating of bone marrow and blood cells, with release of thrombotic and vasoactive substances, and to the hydrolysis of the methylmethacrylate to methacrylate acid. In fact, all these mechanisms probably play a role in one patient or another, judging from the variability in time and extent of the hypotension. (**Ref. 7,** pp. 1226–1227)

175. (C) Meralgia paresthetica is a neuropathy of the lateral femoral cutaneous nerve that is not uncommon during pregnancy. The patient is turned with arms alongside the torso to prevent brachial plexus injuries. Protection of the male genitalia in the prone position is an important consideration, but by far the most important matter is the protection of the eyes. Even slight pressure on the eyeball, for as little as five minutes, may lead to irreversible optic nerve injury and blindness. (**Ref. 36,** pp. 711, 717–718)

176. (A) The radial artery is clearly not a landmark because it forms distally as a branch of the brachial artery. At the elbow, the median nerve lies medial to the brachial artery, between the bicipital aponeurosis and the brachialis muscle. It enters the forearm between the two heads of pronator teres. To block the nerve, the patient's elbow should be extended and the brachial artery palpated 1 to 2 cm above the line joining the two epicondyles. The needle is inserted lateral to the artery passing through the deep fascia. Paresthesia may be obtained or a nerve stimulator used. After aspiration, 0.5 ml is injected initially. If sudden pain should occur, the needle is intraneural and should be withdrawn 1 to 2 mm. If there is no pain, a further 5 ml of local anesthetic solution is injected. (**Ref. 11,** pp. 407–408)

177. (C) The radial nerve lies in the superficial fascia at the wrist, where it divides into its terminal branches. These can all be blocked by subcutaneous infiltration between the radial artery anteriorly and the extensor carpi radialis tendon posteriorly. The radial nerve at this level innervates only the skin. The point of entry of the needle is on a line with the styloid process of the ulna, just lateral to the radial artery, and a band of local anesthetic is injected laterally towards the extensor aspect of the wrist. (**Ref. 11,** p. 411)

178. (D) Kyphoscoliosis causes restrictive, not obstructive lung disease. One of the lungs becomes compressed and the lung volumes are reduced. The thoracic deformity also compresses the pulmonary vessels, which increases pulmonary vascular resistance and eventually leads to right ventricular dysfunction. Chronic hypoxia leads to polycythemia. (**Ref. 46,** pp. 174–189)

108 / 7: Anesthesia for Orthopedic Surgery

179. (A) There are no recognized systemic manifestations of osteoarthritis (OA). OA is the commonest joint disease of humans, affecting 40 to 60 million Americans and is most commonly idiopathic with no predisposing factor apparent. OA is the presenting disease for more than 100,000 total hip and 100,000 knee replacements per year. Excessive stresses on the cartilage causes eventual breakdown of the joint surface, then secondary inflammation and reparative processes lead to osteophyte formation, subchondral erosion, and cyst formation. The clinical manifestations include pain, crepitance, decreased motion, and deformity, most commonly at the hips, knees, feet, and spine. The L_{3-4} level is the spinal level most commonly affected, but the cervical spine may also be involved. Heberden's nodes occur at the distal IP joints and Bouchard's nodes at the PI joints. OA rarely affects the wrists, elbows, or shoulders. (**Ref. 22,** pp. 1692–1698)

180. (B) Rheumatoid arthritis (RA) affects approximately 1% of adults in the United States and is associated with the HLA-DR4 histocompatibility antigen. It affects women 2 to 3 times more frequently than men. Onset of adult RA occurs commonly between the ages of 30 to 50 years. It is a polyarthropathy that can affect any joint, but frequently occurs symmetrically in the hands, wrists, and knees. It may also affect the heart, kidneys, lungs, and eyes. Other joints affected include the cervical spine, the temporomandibular joint, and the cricoarytenoid joints. Cervical spine fusion causing limited range of neck motion and severe pain may occur. Atlantoaxial subluxation may also occur. Surgical stabilization of the neck is usually restricted to symptomatic patients. (**Ref. 46,** p. 10)

181. (B) Approximately 20% to 40% of patients with rheumatoid arthritis have some anterior atlantoaxial subluxation. Posterior subluxation and vertical migration are less common than anterior atlantoaxial subluxation but more dangerous. The atlas can (1) move posteriorly when the odontoid process is destroyed or breaks off the axis or (2) the axis may move vertically within the atlas as a result of the destruction of the lateral atlantoaxial joints or the destruction of bone around the foramen magnum. This can result in severe neurological problems, including quadriplegia. (**Ref. 22,** p. 1651)

182. (B) The cardiac manifestations of rheumatoid arthritis include pericarditis, myocarditis, inflammatory valve involvement, conduction defects, coronary arteritis, and granulomatous aortitis Hematologic manifestations of RA include normocytic hypochromic anemia, eosinophilia, and thrombocytosis. Caplan's syndrome classically occurs in coal miners. It is an interstitial lung disease with diffuse nodular and massive pulmonary fibrosis that occurs in patients with RA and pneumoconiosis. (**Ref. 22,** pp. 1651–1652)

183. (A) Ankylosing spondylitis is relatively common, affecting 1.6% of the population. The disease occurs in both sexes with approximately the same frequency. Cervical spine involvement is variable. The temporomandibular joint may be involved, restricting mouth opening, and cricoarytenoiditis may cause hoarseness or changes in phonation. The signs and symptoms tend to be more severe in men. Cardiac involvement is found in 3.5% of patients with a 25-year history and is higher in patients with a longer history. (**Ref. 46,** p.12)

184. (A) Regional anesthesia can decrease blood loss from THA by 30% to 50%. The same results can be obtained with the use of a hypotensive general anesthetic. Blood flow is increased in the lower extremities.

Spontaneous respiration produces much lower intrathoracic pressures than IPPV and therefore helps to minimize venous bleeding. (**Ref. 46,** pp. 70–72)

185. (C) Following THA the incidence of DVT is 40% to 60% and the incidence of pulmonary embolism is 2% to 3%. Fatal pulmonary thromboemboli have been reported in 0.3% to 2.4% of patients undergoing hip arthroplasty and in 4% to 7% after surgery for hip fractures. Epidural and spinal anesthesia significantly reduce the incidence of DVT and PE after operative fixation of the hip and total hip or knee arthroplasty. (**Ref. 46,** pp. 72–78)

186. (A) The following may contribute to the antithromboembolic effects of regional anesthesia. Local anesthetics, especially the amides (1) may reduce the adhesion of the leukocytes to the vessel walls; (2) cause higher resting levels of plasminogen; (3) result in increased capacity to release plasminogen activators; (4) increase blood flow to the lower extremities. (**Ref. 46,** pp. 72–78)

187. (**B**) Intraoperative hypotension and cardiovascular collapse have occurred with cemented femoral shaft placement. Venous embolism may occur when the cement and the femoral component are forced into the reamed femoral shaft. Emboli may include bone fragments, air, clots, and methylmethacrylate liquid monomer. These emboli may cause release of tissue thromboplastin and platelet and fibrin aggregation in the pulmonary circulation. Platelet aggregation can lead to the release of vasoactive substances, which leads to vasodilation and hypotension. Methylmethacrylate is supplied as a liquid (monomer) and a powder (polymer). Unpolymerized liquid monomer is volatile and can be absorbed into the bloodstream where it may act as a direct vasodilator. Particles of methylmethacrylate may be absorbed and cause direct pulmonary injury. Decreases in PaO_2 occurring at the time of the placement of the femoral component are most likely related to pulmonary embolism, not to vasodilation. (**Ref. 32,** p. 1964; **Ref. 46,** pp. 355–358)

188. (**B**) Pressure on the ulnar nerve or traction of the C_8-T_1 roots of the brachial plexus at the first rib results in numbness over the distribution of the ulnar nerve in the hand. Pressure below the head of the fibula results in paresis of the common peroneal nerve and foot drop. Pressure over the anterior iliac crest leads to paresis of the lateral cutaneous nerve of thigh (meralgia paresthetica) and numbness of the lateral thigh. Pressure on the posterior aspect of the upper arm, where the nerve spirals around the back of the humerus, may cause paresis of the radial nerve and result in wrist drop. (**Ref. 32,** p. 1954)

189. (**C**) A certain degree of lung dysfunction occurs in all patients following all long-bone fracture, but clinically significant FES develops in only 10% to 15%. Mortality associated with FES is 10% to 20%. The incidence of FES increases with fractures of the pelvis and with multiple traumatic fractures. (**Ref. 46,** pp. 357–358; **Ref. 32,** p. 1964)

190. (**A**) In FES there is an increase in the levels of free fatty acids, serum triglycerides, and serum lipase activity, as well as frank fat

globules that may have entered the venous system through torn veins. These globules may then lodge in the pulmonary vascular bed causing V/Q mismatch and a decreased PaO_2. (**Ref. 46, pp. 357–358**)

191. (D) Mortality after hip surgery is high. Although regional anesthesia is believed by some to be preferable to general anesthesia, there is no conclusive evidence to support this. Long-term survival rates show no advantage of regional anesthesia over general anesthesia. Postoperative hypoxemia is significantly greater and lasts longer after general anesthesia than after regional anesthesia. Regional anesthesia may have some other advantages, but improved mortality is not one of them. (**Ref. 46, pp. 90–93**)

192. (A) Patients with spinal curves of greater than 60° often have the pulmonary respiratory pattern of restrictive, not obstructive, disease. Scoliosis is graded by a system using a measurement called the Cobb angle. The greater the angle, the more severe the spinal curvature. In patients with idiopathic scoliosis, the Cobb angle can be correlated with pulmonary dysfunction. Patients with angles less than 50° usually have no respiratory abnormality. If the angle is greater than 100°, the patient may have marked signs and symptoms of respiratory failure. (**Ref. 46, pp. 11, 174–176**)

193. (B) Scoliotic deformities can affect respiratory mechanics, gas exchange, pulmonary vasculature, and the chemical regulation of ventilation. Ventilation-perfusion (V/Q) mismatch is common and is a significant problem. As the V/Q abnormalities worsen, ventilatory demands increase. Inability to meet these demands eventually results in hypercapnia and respiratory failure. (**Ref. 46, pp. 179–180**)

194. (C) In patients with untreated scoliosis, death usually occurs by age 45. Cor pulmonale or respiratory failure accounts for 60% of deaths. Postoperative mechanical ventilation is likely to be required for patients with a vital capacity less than 40% of that which was predicted. A loud second heart sound, as evidence of pulmonary hypertension, is not unusual in severe cases. Postoperatively pulmonary function often deteriorates acutely. Vital capacity decreases by 40% and the alveolar–arterial oxygen gradient increases by 50%. These changes may require 7 to 10 days to resolve. Significant improvement in respiratory function is unlikely and rarely exceeds a 10% increase in vital capacity one year postoperatively. (**Ref. 46,** pp. 179–180)

195. **(E)** Deliberate hypotensive anesthesia (also called induced or controlled hypotension) first described in 1946, has been shown to decrease blood loss, operating time, and the need for transfusions. Hemodilution involves withdrawing 20% to 30% of the blood volume at the beginning of surgery and replacing it at a 3:1 ratio with Ringer's lactate solution. The preserved blood is replaced toward the end of the procedure with a simultaneous diuresis of the now excess fluid. (**Ref. 46,** pp. 20–45)

196. **(A)** A reduction in anterior spinal artery blood flow produces ischemia of the anterior regions of the cord, which may result in motor weakness or paralysis of the lower extremities. In some cases, this may occur without observed alterations in somatosensory-evoked potentials. No patient has been neurologically intact intraoperatively and then had a neurologic deficit postoperatively. The wake-up test tests motor function only. In the classic wake-up test a nitrous oxide-narcotic relaxant technique is used for anesthesia. No potent anesthetic vapors are given, since these may delay wake-up for as much as 30 minutes. Narcotic or neuromuscular blockade antagonists are not used intraoperatively since they may cause overly sudden alertness and dangerously excessive movement on the operating table. The shorter acting muscle relaxants like vecuronium and atracurium are useful in this regard. Spinal cord function tests may be performed on any patient undergoing major scoliosis surgery, although a wake-up test may be difficult to perform on young children or mentally deficient patients. (**Ref. 32,** p. 1959)

197. **(A)** After the release of a tourniquet, there is a rise in acid metabolites entering the circulation. Plasma bicarbonates buffer the acid metabolites, and this results in an elevation of $PaCO_2$. As the elevated $PaCO_2$ circulates centrally, it stimulates the respiratory center and may result in increases in respiratory rate or depth. Deflation of a tourniquet may cause an acute decrease in SVR, central venous and arterial pressures. The resultant fall in blood pressure can be profound, and even cardiac arrest has resulted. Core temperature may decrease by approximately 0.5 to 1.0°C on cuff deflation. (**Ref. 32,** pp. 1962–1964; **Ref. 46,** pp. 89–90)

198. **(A)** Evidence suggests that mitochondrial PO_2 falls to zero within 6 minutes of inflating a tourniquet, after which time anaerobic metabolism begins. Decrease of nicotinamide adenine dinucleotide and creatinine phosphate stores in muscle occurs over the next 30 to 60 minutes. Cellular acidosis (pH < 6.5) rapidly ensues. Hypoxia and acidosis result in the release of myoglobin, intracellular enzymes, and potassium.

    Thromboxane is released locally with disruption of endothelial integrity. Tissue edema develops if tourniquets are inflated for more than 60 minutes. Cellular ischemic changes are reversible after 2 hours. Within 30 minutes of inflation, nerve conduction ceases and neurological problems may occur after inflation for longer than 2 hours. In clinical practice tourniquets should be deflated every 90 to 120 minutes. (**Ref. 46,** pp. 1962–1964)

199. **(B)** $PaCO_2$ may increase by 20 mm Hg and pH can decrease by 0.2 units, lactate levels increase, serum potassium may increase by 0.5 mMol/L. After one hour of leg ischemia time, the cooled limb will lower body temperature by approximately 0.7°C. Possible causes of decreasing temperature include the cooling effect of blood from the ischemic extremity flowing centrally, cooling of systemic blood flowing through the ischemic extremity, and reactive hyperemia after tourniquet deflation, with increased heat loss from the extremity. (**Ref. 32,** pp. 1962–1964)

200. **(B)** Nerve damage is thought to be primarily due to pressure and to anatomic distortion at the edge of the cuff and not primarily to ischemia. Tourniquet pain is typically an ill-defined aching or burning pain that usually appears 45 to 60 minutes after inflation of the tourniquet. It is probably mediated by small, unmyelinated C fibers and is relieved by deflation of the tourniquet for 10 to 15 minutes, after which time the cuff may be reinflated. (**Ref. 32,** pp. 1962–1964; **Ref. 46,** pp. 89–90)

8

Anesthesia for Gynecological Surgery

DIRECTIONS (Questions 201–214): Each of the questions or incomplete statements below is followed by five suggested answers or completions. Select the **one** that is best in each case.

201. Nerve injury from the use of stirrups for lithotomy position is most likely to involve the
    A. pudendal nerve
    B. posterior tibial nerve
    C. obturator nerve
    D. common peroneal nerve
    E. femoral nerve

202. The nerve supply to the vulva originates from
    A. S_2, S_3, S_4
    B. L_5, S_1, S_2
    C. the genitofemoral nerve
    D. the medial cutaneous nerve of the thigh
    E. the sciatic nerve

203. Common presenting signs and symptoms of an ectopic pregnancy include all of the following EXCEPT
   A. pain
   B. abnormal vaginal bleeding
   C. abdominal tenderness
   D. thrombocytopenia
   E. palpable pelvic mass

204. A patient undergoing a TAH–BSO under regional anesthesia experiences a total epidural block. Respiratory depression ensues due to
   A. phrenic nerve block
   B. shifting of the CO_2 response curve to the right
   C. shifting of the CO_2 response curve to the left
   D. over sedation with propofol
   E. medullary ischemia due to hypotension and decreased cardiac output

205. When instituting the Trendelenburg position, all the following physiologic changes may be expected EXCEPT
   A. increased inspiratory pressures with controlled ventilation
   B. ventilation/perfusion ratio changes
   C. increased right ventricular stress
   D. increased left ventricular stress
   E. minimal changes in cardiac output and mean arterial pressure

206. A patient receives 0.2 mg of methylergonovine intravenously following an elective abortion. All the following consequences may occur EXCEPT
   A. seizures
   B. retinal detachment
   C. hypotension
   D. nausea and vomiting
   E. cerebrovascular accident

116 / 8: Anesthesia for Gynecological Surgery

207. When performing cervical dilation and curettage or evacuation, a paracervical blockade
  A. prevents discomfort from the most painful portion of the surgery
  B. prevents discomfort from uterine curettage
  C. prevents early detection of uterine perforation
  D. prevents hypotension
  E. leads to uterine atony

208. A 50-year-old woman has a subarachnoid block for a Marshall-Marchetti-Krantz procedure for urinary incontinence. A postdural puncture headache (PDPH) occurs on postoperative day 2. True statements include all of the following EXCEPT
  A. enforced flat bedrest could have prevented the PDPH
  B. success rates for the first epidural blood patch are 90% to 95%
  C. repeat blood patch, if needed, has a success rate of 90% to 95%
  D. the patient may also complain of diplopia and photophobia
  E. appropriate conservative measures include forced fluid intake of 3 liters/day, analgesics, tight abdominal binders, and intravenous caffeine

209. Carbon dioxide laser vaporization (fulguration) of vulvar intraepithelial neoplasias entails all the following risks EXCEPT
  A. thermal injury from reflected laser light
  B. carbon dioxide embolus
  C. ignition of operative drapes
  D. retinal injury
  E. viral inoculation from inhalation of particulates in the laser plume

210. Which of the following statements are false regarding a patient scheduled for a debulking procedure for a large pelvic malignancy?
  A. the patient should be considered as having a full stomach
  B. the patient does not require left uterine displacement to prevent caval compression
  C. the patient is at an increased risk for pulmonary embolus
  D. the patient will likely encounter respiratory compromise in the Trendelenburg position
  E. the patient may be malnourished

211. A patient is scheduled to undergo TAH–BSO, omentectomy, partial small bowel resection, and splenectomy for pelvic carcinomatosis. Anesthetic considerations include
    A. use of low-flow techniques to minimize heat loss
    B. abdominal distention from nitrous oxide
    C. hypotension from major blood loss and fluid shifts
    D. development of coagulopathy
    E. avoidance of a combined epidural–general anesthetic technique

212. A patient receives a subarachnoid block with 75 mg of hyperbaric lidocaine for a cone biopsy. Major factors affecting the level of anesthesia achieved include
    A. dosage of lidocaine
    B. the patient's age
    C. the patient's height
    D. the technique of injection
    E. the anatomic configuration of the spinal column

213. Excellent perineal anesthesia may be achieved with a caudal block. Anatomic considerations when entering the sacral canal include all of the following EXCEPT
    A. frequent variations in sacral anatomy
    B. termination of the dural sac is lower in adults than in children
    C. the sacral hiatus is covered by the posterior sacrococcygeal ligament
    D. the absence of a sacral hiatus on 5% of patients
    E. the angle of needle insertion for males is almost parallel to the skin whereas the angle is slightly deeper in females

118 / 8: Anesthesia for Gynecological Surgery

214. Which of the following statements is NOT correct regarding a patient undergoing a vaginal hysterectomy under subarachnoid block with a level at T_6?
   A. this level is needed to block painful peritoneal sensations from uterine traction
   B. a large bore IV should be in place
   C. a type and antibody screen should be performed preoperatively
   D. excessive uterine size, intraabdominal adhesions, or suspicion of intrapelvic malignancy may cause the surgeon to abandon the transvaginal approach
   E. severe bradycardia may occur with uterine traction due to blockade of the cardiac sympathetic innervation

---

DIRECTIONS (Questions 215–229): For each of the questions or incomplete statements below, **one** or **more** of the answers given is correct. Select
   A. if only 1, 2, and 3 are correct
   B. if only 1 and 3 are correct
   C. if only 2 and 4 are correct
   D. if only 4 is correct
   E. if all are correct

---

215. The pudendal nerve provides
   1. motor fibers to the external anal sphincter
   2. sensory fibers to the cervix
   3. sensory fibers to the labia or scrotum
   4. autonomic innervation to the bladder

216. Complication rates from therapeutic dilation and evacuation directly correlate with
   1. gestational age
   2. anesthetic technique
   3. experience of the surgeon
   4. use of a paracervical block

217. Before insertion of a Verres (insufflation) needle for a diagnostic laparoscopy, the anesthesiologist should
   1. ensure adequate muscle relaxation
   2. hold ventilation

3. empty the patient's stomach
4. place the patient in reverse Trendelenburg position

218. Appropriate treatment for a massive CO_2 embolus during diagnostic laparoscopy includes
    1. stopping further insufflation
    2. restoring effective cardiac output
    3. placing central venous catheter and attempting to withdraw air
    4. placing the patient in a left lateral head-down position

219. Patients undergoing suction curettage for a complete hydatidiform mole are likely (>25%) to present with
    1. anemia
    2. preeclampsia
    3. hyperemesis
    4. hyperthyroidism

220. During a diagnostic laparoscopy the patient's end tidal CO_2 increases from 38 mm Hg to 42 mm Hg over a ten-minute period. Concurrent events are likely to be
    1. an increase in peak inspiratory pressure
    2. a 3°C rise in core temperature
    3. mild increase in blood pressure
    4. multifocal PVCs

221. During laparoscopy the end tidal CO_2 level quickly falls from 38 to 18. Concurrent events are likely to be
    1. hypotension
    2. an increase in dead space
    3. arterial desaturation
    4. a mill-wheel murmur

222. When changing from the lithotomy position to the supine position, the patient's legs should first be brought together in the sagittal plane and then lowered slowly in order to
    1. avoid sudden hypotension
    2. avoid premature patient stimulation
    3. minimize stress on the lumbar spine
    4. prevent the aortacaval syndrome

8: Anesthesia for Gynecological Surgery

223. Anesthetic management of a ruptured ectopic pregnancy includes
    1. securing the airway
    2. the use of O-negative blood
    3. several large-bore IVs
    4. immediate surgery

224. Following TAH–BSO and omentectomy as well as chemotherapy for ovarian cancer, the patient complains of left-sided upper lateral thigh pain and paresthesias. Other findings may include
    1. these complaints may worsen with hip extension
    2. her left leg is significantly weaker than the right
    3. her course of chemotherapy included *cis*-platinum
    4. her complaints may worsen with hip flexion

225. The post-dural puncture headache is usually characterized by
    1. its immediate appearance following dural puncture
    2. accompanying nuchal rigidity
    3. a mainly bitemporal location
    4. a postural component

226. Nausea and vomiting are common complications of outpatient laparoscopy. Which of the following statements is (are) true?
    1. low doses of droperidol used prophylactically have been shown to decrease the incidence of nausea and vomiting postoperatively
    2. these complications are especially of concern in patients with a history of motion sickness
    3. emesis is a leading cause of unanticipated hospital admission
    4. surgery around the time of menses leads to a fourfold increase in the incidence of nausea and vomiting

227. A 32-year-old woman presents for a cone biopsy. Her last menstrual period was 21 days ago. As her anesthesiologist you
    1. must insist that a pregnancy test be done
    2. must use a regional anesthetic technique
    3. know that a pregnancy test will accurately detect pregnancy at this stage
    4. feel that a pregnancy test is not mandatory

228. Carbon dioxide is used to insufflate the abdomen for laparoscopy because
  1. it is nonflammable
  2. it is highly soluble in blood
  3. it is quickly absorbed by the peritoneal surfaces
  4. it does not cause referred pain to the scapula

229. Inspiratory pressures rise from 25 to 40 mm Hg in an obese patient undergoing laparoscopy. It is important for the anesthesiologist to
  1. provide an adequate depth of anesthesia
  2. provide muscle relaxation
  3. reduce the degree of Trendelenburg positioning and/or advise the surgeon to release some of the CO_2 from the abdomen
  4. rule out tension pneumothorax

Anesthesia for Gynecological Surgery

Answers and Discussion

The authors have made every effort to thoroughly verify the answers to the questions that appear on the preceding pages. As in any text, however, some inaccuracies and ambiguities may occur. If in doubt, please consult the indicated reference. When no page number(s) are cited, the reference is to a journal article or to a refresher course lecture that should be read in its entirety.

The Editors

201. (D) The common peroneal nerve may be injured in the lithotomy position by compression between the fibula and the stirrups or by inward rotation of the leg at the thigh causing the common peroneal nerve to be stretched around the head of the fibula. The ensuing neurologic deficit will be a "foot drop" (i.e., inability to flex the foot at the ankle). The injury is usually limited in duration but may be permanent. (**Ref. 36,** p. 712)

202. (A) The pudendal nerve arises from spinal nerves S_2, S_3, and S_4. It ends by dividing into the perineal nerve and the dorsal nerve of the penis/clitoris. Gynecological surgery involving the perineum or rectum requires blocking these sacral nerve roots. This may be accomplished with a subarachnoid block or with an epidural block, using either the lumbar or caudal approach. (**Ref. 18, p. 1149**)

203. (D) The incidence of tubal ectopic pregnancy has dramatically increased to approximately 1/100 pregnancies. The development of more sensitive pregnancy tests in conjunction with ultrasonography has improved the early detection of small ectopic pregnancies. Despite this, it is important to realize that the presenting signs and symptoms are often nonspecific. Tubal ectopic pregnancies may rupture without warning and require urgent resuscitation and surgical exploration and repair. (**Ref. 36, p. 2121**)

204. (E) High thoracic sensory levels from spinal or epidural blocks do not affect blood gases, tidal volumes, or inspiratory volumes but may decrease expiratory volumes and pressures. Even midcervical levels will not grossly affect the function of the phrenic nerves. The respiratory depression seen from high spinals or total epidurals is due to the effects of hypotension and decreased cardiac output on the medulla and not to the effect of local anesthetic on the respiratory center. (**Ref. 5, #136, p. 3**)

205. (D) Cephalad displacement of the diaphragm in Trendelenburg position and obstruction of its inspiratory stroke increases the work of breathing in spontaneously ventilating patients and increases inspiratory pressures during controlled ventilation. Ventilation–perfusion ratios worsen because of gravitational increases in blood flow to the poorly ventilated apices of the lungs. Head-down tilt only minimally increases cardiac output and mean arterial pressure. This coupled with deteriorating pulmonary function, however, increases right ventricular stress. The Trendelenburg position should be used with caution in patients with pulmonary disease or right ventricular compromise. This position should also be used with caution in patients with intracranial pathology resulting from increased intravascular congestion and increased intracranial pressure. (**Ref. 7, pp. 715–716**)

206. (C) Methylergonovine (methergine) should never be given if there is any indication that a cerebrovascular accident or a retinal detachment is threatening. In addition, seizures may be triggered by this drug. Nausea and vomiting in the awake patient may be due to direct central nervous system stimulation. Methylergonovine should be used with caution in patients with coronary artery disease, hypertension, and preeclampsia. (**Ref. 36,** p. 2107)

207. (A) The most stimulating part of a D&C or a D&E is the cervical dilation. This discomfort is managed quite well by a paracervical block. A paracervical block does not, however, anesthetize the uterine fundus and as a result curettage may be uncomfortable. The majority of therapeutic abortions are performed under paracervical block with or without IV sedation because this allows for the rapid detection of uterine perforation. The patient is able to complain of sudden, acute abdominal pain. In addition, average blood loss from a D&E is higher when general anesthesia is used due to uterine relaxation or atony from the volatile agents. (**Ref. 36,** pp. 2114–2117)

208. (A) Bed rest may control the symptoms of PDPH after it occurs. However, it does not prevent but merely delays the onset of PDPH. Conservative measures include abdominal binders, injection of sterile saline into the epidural space, forced fluid intake, caffeine, and analgesics. Epidural blood patches are the most efficacious treatment for PDPH when the problem is not self-limited. They have a success rate of 90% to 95% with the first injection and may be repeated in 24 hours with a similar success rate. (**Ref. 11,** pp. 246–247)

209. (B) Any operative laser use entails certain risks to both the patient and the hospital staff. Sudden movements by the patient can cause the laser beam to strike an unintended area, resulting in fire or thermal injury. All operating room personnel should wear certified protective goggles. Typical eye care for the patient involves the use of eye pads moistened with saline solution, as well as protective goggles. The use of special laser surgical masks to trap virus-containing particles is recommended. (**Ref. 36,** pp. 2111–2112)

210. (B) Patients undergoing debulking procedures have varying degrees of small bowel obstruction due to tumor mass and should be considered to have full stomachs. Any large pelvic mass may compress the vena cava, and left uterine displacement will help to prevent hypotension. All patients with malignancies may have a

hypercoaguable state predisposing them to pulmonary embolus both in the intraoperative and postoperative periods. Many cancer patients suffer from cachexia, resulting in hypoalbuminemia and changes in protein binding ability. (**Ref. 36,** p. 2126)

211. **(E)** A combined epidural–general technique is often indicated for these procedures—the sympathetic blockade from the epidural promotes bowel contraction allowing for an easier dissection. Nitrous oxide should be avoided or discontinued if distended loops of bowel are present. The epidural may also be beneficial postoperatively for pain control. (**Ref. 36,** p. 2128)

212. **(A)** The major factors affecting the level of anesthesia achieved with a spinal anesthetic include the position of the patient, the baricity of the local anesthetic solution used, and the volume of drug injected. (**Ref. 32,** p. 1393)

213. **(B)** The sacral hiatus is formed by the failure of the laminae of S_5 to fuse in the midline. The width and size of this bony defect can vary widely and may be absent in 5% of patients, precluding a caudal approach. The sacral hiatus is covered by the sacrococcygeal ligament or membrane, which is the functional counterpart to the ligamentum flavum. The angle of the sacral canal is slightly steeper in women than in men. The termination of the dural sac is at S_2 in adults and at S_{3-4} in early childhood. (**Ref. 32,** pp. 1379–1399)

214. **(E)** Severe bradycardia may result from uterine traction caused by a vagal response. Treatment is with intravenous atropine. Bradycardia during spinal anesthesia results from the level of the block extending to T_1–T_4 dermatomes and blocking the cardioaccelerator nerves. Sudden major blood loss may occur while freeing up the uterus from a vascular pedicle or unsuspected intraabdominal adhesions. For this reason large-bore IV access is a requirement. Blood, typed and screened for antibodies, must be available preoperatively, and a type and screen should always be available postoperatively. (**Ref. 36,** p. 2118)

215. **(B)** The pudendal nerve supplies sensation to the lower half of the anal and perianal skin and to the posterior surface of the scrotum/labia and penis/clitoris. It supplies muscular branches

to the external anal sphincter and the superficial and deep perineal muscles, the bulbospongiosus, ischiocavernosus, sphincter urethrae, and the levator ani. (**Ref. 18,** p. 1149)

216. **(B)** Complication rates from therapeutic dilation and evacuation do correlate directly with surgical experience and gestational age. While anesthetic technique does not alter complication rates, most of these procedures are performed under a paracervical block to allow for rapid detection of uterine perforation. (**Ref. 36,** p. 2116)

217. **(A)** A momentary hold on ventilation and a relaxed and immobile abdomen is required for insertion of the Verres needle to avoid bringing the needle in contact with the stomach or other viscera. Sudden increases in intraabdominal pressure from coughing or straining may result in organ perforation or in the laceration of a major blood vessel in the pelvis. (**Ref. 36,** pp. 2128–2133)

218. **(E)** Massive carbon dioxide embolus during laparoscopy is a rare but potentially catastrophic event. Left lateral head-down position will help to trap gas in the right ventricle rather than allowing it to go into the pulmonary outflow tract. A central venous catheter placed into the right atrium may be used to aspirate gas and lessen the mechanical obstruction to cardiac output. During a state of cardiovascular collapse, the patient should be supported with 100% oxygen and vasopressors to restore effective cardiac output. (**Ref. 36,** p. 2132)

219. **(A)** A hydatidiform mole is a neoplastic growth resulting from deranged placental growth. Anemia is present in over 50% of cases due to abnormal vaginal bleeding. Preeclampsia and hyperemesis are also present in 27% and 26% of patients, respectively. Hyperthyroidism and pulmonary trophoblastic emboli are rare but life-threatening complications. (**Ref. 36,** p. 2116)

220. **(B)** Mild increases in end-tidal CO_2 are expected during laparoscopy due to intraperitoneal uptake of the insufflated carbon dioxide. This can almost always be compensated for by using higher minute volumes in ventilated patients. Mild hypertension

may also occur due to stimulation from peritoneal stretch and the mild respiratory acidosis. (**Ref. 36,** p. 2130)

221. (E) One of the goals of anesthesia for laparoscopic surgery is the rapid detection of a gas embolus. Events usually include the sudden onset of hypotension, tachycardia, and pulmonary edema. A holosystolic and diastolic mill-wheel murmur can result from foaming of the blood within the right heart and pulmonary outflow tract. Capnography usually shows a sudden drop in end-tidal CO_2 due to the acute increase in physiologic dead space. (**Ref. 36,** p. 2132)

222. (B) When going from the lithotomy to the supine position, legs are first brought together in the midline while elevated and then lowered slowly to allow for gradual accommodation to the increase in venous capacitance, thus avoiding sudden decreases in venous return and hypotension. Bringing the legs together before lowering them minimizes torsional stress on the lumbar spine that would occur if the legs were lowered independently. (**Ref. 7,** p. 712)

223. (E) Much like a ruptured aortic aneurysm, treatment of a ruptured ectopic pregnancy revolves around rapid fluid resuscitation and concurrent, immediate surgery to control the bleeding. Type O-negative blood may be used if type-specific blood is not available. Large-bore IV access is a must, along with pressurized infusion devices. (**Ref. 36,** p. 2122)

224. (B) Isolated pain, burning, or tingling in the upper lateral thigh is rarely caused by anything other than meralgia paresthetica (entrapment of the lateral femoral cutaneous nerve). This nerve has no motor fibers so the symptoms should be purely sensory. The symptoms are usually mild and often alleviated by hip flexion and exacerbated by hip extension. Sensory action potentials may show a conduction delay or be absent. EMG should reveal no abnormalities of the quadriceps muscle or the femoral nerve. *cis*-Platinum is an active chemotherapeutic agent against ovarian carcinoma. It has the potential to produce renal tubular dysfunction, ototoxicity, myelosuppression, and peripheral neuropathies that may be severe. (**Ref. 9,** p. 1525; **Ref. 36,** p. 2132)

225. **(D)** Clinical features of a PDPH include (1) onset several hours to 1–2 days post puncture, (2) bifrontal and occipital location, (3) aggravated by the upright position and dramatically relieved by the supine position, and (4) associated symptoms include nausea, photophobia and in severe cases diplopia and cranial nerve palsies due to traction on the cranial nerves. (**Ref. 11,** p. 246)

226. **(E)** Uncontrolled nausea and vomiting are major problems following ambulatory surgery, not only because they lead to unanticipated admission but because treatment may result in prolonged somnolence. Pain, the use of narcotic analgesics, obesity, sudden position changes, history of motion sickness, site of surgery, and timing of surgery around menses all may contribute to increasing the incidence of nausea and vomiting. Choice of induction agents may influence the incidence of nausea and vomiting. Ketamine and etomidate result in more nausea and vomiting than the barbiturates, which in turn are associated with a higher incidence than propofol. Epidural anesthesia may also be appropriate for certain laparoscopies and is associated with a significantly lower incidence of postoperative nausea and vomiting. Many studies have found droperidol in doses ranging from 0.25 to 0.625 mg to be an effective prophylactic antiemetic in the outpatient population. (**Ref. 47,** pp. 389–397)

227. **(D)** The American College of Obstetrics and Gynecology (ACOG) does not require mandatory pregnancy testing of all females of childbearing age but does require testing if there is any question after a thorough history or in the event of suggestive signs or symptoms. The ACOG standard, however, also identifies the need for each institution to have a policy regarding the determination of pregnancy. Whatever the institutional policy—whether it views a totally negative history and physical as adequate, or whether pregnancy tests are required for all female patients between the ages of 12 and 50—it should be adhered to rigorously. (**Ref. 47,** pp. 62–63)

228. **(A)** Carbon dioxide is nonflammable and quickly absorbed by peritoneal tissues. It is highly soluble in blood, therefore it rapidly goes into solution in blood vessels should an embolus occur. Although it is rapidly taken up and removed, residual intraperitoneal

carbon dioxide does exert pressure on the diaphragm, resulting in referred pain to the scapula. (**Ref. 36,** pp. 2128–2132)

229. **(E)** Increases in inspiratory pressures are common during laparoscopy, especially in obese patients. If the pressures become unacceptably high, especially if accompanied by decreases in oxygen saturation, changes in positioning and carbon dioxide insufflation pressures may be warranted and tension pneumothorax due to barotrauma must be ruled out. Pulmonary barotrauma is defined as extraalveolar air due to lung damage from changes in intrathoracic pressure. Tension pneumothorax results when pleural gas is under greater than ambient pressure. This leads to displacement of the mediastinal structures, decreased venous return to the heart, cardiovascular collapse and an essentially complete inability to ventilate the patient. Insertion of a 14-gauge needle into the second intercostal space may confirm the diagnosis and decompress the tension pneumothorax, although a tube thoracostomy (chest tube placement) may be required for more prolonged decompression. (**Ref. 36,** p. 2130; **Ref. 32,** p. 2195)

9
Anesthesia for Ear, Nose, and Throat and Oral Surgery

DIRECTIONS (Questions 230–239): Each of the questions or incomplete statements below is followed by five suggested answers or completions. Select the **one** that is best in each case.

230. Which of the following muscles tenses the vocal cords?
    A. cricoarytenoid
    B. cricothyroid
    C. thyroarytenoid
    D. thyrohyoid
    E. interarytenoid

231. The principal adductor of the vocal cords is
    A. thyroepiglottic
    B. aryepiglottic
    C. lateral cricoarytenoid
    D. interarytenoid
    E. cricothyroid

232. Which one of the following muscles is a depressor of the larynx?
    A. mylohyoid
    B. cricothyroid
    C. thyrohyoid
    D. sternothyroid
    E. digastric

233. The anterior two-third of the tongue is innervated by the
    A. glossopharyngeal nerve
    B. mandibular nerve
    C. maxillary nerve
    D. vagus nerve
    E. superior laryngeal nerve

234. The most important role in preventing aspiration during swallowing is played by the
    A. epiglottis
    B. tongue
    C. true vocal folds
    D. aryepiglottic folds
    E. false vocal folds

235. The vocal cord function that is usually affected by minor damage is
    A. adduction
    B. tensor action
    C. abduction
    D. rotation
    E. phonation

236. The commonest cause of airway compromise following surgery in the anterior and/or lateral portion of the neck is
    A. unilateral severing of the recurrent laryngeal nerve
    B. bilateral injury to the recurrent laryngeal nerves
    C. hematoma of the neck
    D. loss of blood supply to the recurrent laryngeal nerve
    E. tracheal collapse

237. Management of an endotracheal fire includes all of the following EXCEPT
   A. extubation and mask ventilation
   B. removal of oxygen source
   C. extubation and reintubation
   D. suctioning of the debris from the airway
   E. rigid bronchoscopy

238. The hazards of laser surgery include all of the following EXCEPT
   A. corneal damage
   B. retinal damage
   C. airway fires
   D. fetal abnormalities in pregnant OR personnel
   E. hemorrhage

239. The following precautions should be used during laser surgery to prevent airway fires EXCEPT
   A. ventilating the patient by using a jet ventilator instead of an endotracheal tube
   B. using a laser tube instead of an ordinary ET tube
   C. using a metal ET tube
   D. Using a 50% N_2O–50% O_2 mixture during the procedure
   E. using a heliox mixture to minimize flammability and to optimize ventilation through the stenotic area

DIRECTIONS (Questions 240–256): For each of the questions or incomplete answers below, **one** or **more** of the answers or completions are correct. Select

- **A.** if only 1, 2, and 3 are correct
- **B.** if only 1 and 3 are correct
- **C.** if only 2 and 4 are correct
- **D.** if only 4 is correct
- **E.** if all are correct

240. A 24-year-old female is 8 hours post a mandibular advancement procedure. Her jaws are wired shut. She was doing well, when she complained of nausea and retched. Within 2 to 3 minutes she became apneic, developed bradycardia, and very shortly thereafter suffered a cardiac arrest. The airway is best managed by
    1. oral intubation after cutting the wires
    2. mask ventilation to protect integrity of the mandible
    3. tracheotomy
    4. nasal fiberoptic intubation

241. The following statement(s) is (are) true about patients with sleep apnea
    1. they may be treated with continuous positive airway pressure (CPAP) for the obstructive component
    2. they benefit from sedation during minor surgical procedures
    3. mask ventilation will be difficult after induction of anesthesia
    4. tracheal intubation is not usually difficult

242. The Klippel–Feil syndrome is associated with
    1. cervical vertebral fusion
    2. Sprengel's deformity
    3. low hairline
    4. short extremities

243. During septoplasty the surgeon infiltrates lidocaine with epinephrine. The risk of cardiac arrhythmia is increased if the anesthesiologist uses
    1. vecuronium
    2. halothane
    3. atracurium
    4. pancuronium

244. The complications of tracheotomy include
    1. hemorrhage
    2. tracheal stenosis
    3. tracheoesophageal fistula
    4. massive air embolism

245. For awake intubation of a morbidly obese patient, the important steps to follow are
    1. heavy sedation
    2. topical anesthesia of the oral and nasal pharynx
    3. transtracheal epinephrine to decrease bleeding
    4. bilateral superior laryngeal nerve block

246. Anesthetic considerations in a patient with severe rheumatoid arthritis include
    1. temporomandibular joint (TMJ) arthritis limiting mouth opening
    2. coronary artery disease
    3. complications of steroid therapy
    4. obstructive pulmonary disease

247. A patient with hereditary angioedema
    1. suffers from episodic painless edema of the upper airway
    2. benefits from regional technique when possible, thereby avoiding tracheal intubation
    3. benefits from prophylactic treatment with danazol
    4. decreases the chances of developing an episode with a transfusion of fresh frozen plasma (FFP)

248. A 28-year-old male undergoing septoplasty develops hypertension, tachycardia, and PVCs
  1. he may benefit from changing the inhalation agent from isoflurane to halothane
  2. local injection of epinephrine may have caused these hemodynamic changes
  3. the commonest cause is an allergic reaction to lidocaine
  4. the local use of cocaine may have contributed to the hemodynamic changes

249. Nasotracheal intubation has the following complications:
  1. infection
  2. sore throat
  3. excessive bleeding
  4. tracheal stenosis

250. Post-intubation laryngeal edema can be managed by
  1. IV Decadron
  2. racemic epinephrine treatment
  3. assisted ventilation
  4. PEEP

251. The difference(s) in upper airway anatomy between children and adults is (are)
  1. children have relatively large tongue
  2. the adult larynx is situated more cephalad and anterior
  3. in children the narrowest part of the airway is at the level of the cricoid cartilage
  4. in adults the epiglottis is long and stiff when compared to that of children

252. Following complete preoxygenation, if intubation is difficult
  1. a 70-kg healthy patient will desaturate within 5 minutes
  2. a 4-kg infant will desaturate within 5 minutes
  3. a 150-kg adult will have enough reserve for about 8 minutes because of the large size
  4. a 70-kg healthy adult has enough reserve for 8 to 10 minutes

253. In a patient with acromegaly, intubation may be difficult because of
    1. protruding mandible
    2. macroglossia
    3. enlarged epiglottis
    4. thickening of the vocal cords

254. Management of a patient with an anterior mediastinal mass includes the following:
    1. they may benefit from irradiation to debulk the tumor prior to surgery
    2. rapid sequence induction with succinylcholine is the method of choice
    3. arterial line and Swan–Ganz catheterization from the femoral approach may be necessary
    4. if the endotracheal tube is correctly placed, ventilation is not a problem

255. After induction of anesthesia using pentothal and succinylcholine, the patient for nonemergent cesarean section is found to be impossible to intubate. The safe options include
    1. awakening the patient and doing fiberoptic intubation
    2. continuing with general anesthesia with mask under cricoid pressure
    3. obtaining patient consent and attempting a continuous epidural
    4. repositioning the airway, administering a nondepolarizing muscle relaxant and calling for help from other endoscopists

256. Anesthetic considerations in a patient with severe rheumatoid arthritis include
    1. atlantoaxial instability
    2. micrognathia
    3. cricoarytenoid arthritis
    4. severe chronic obstructive pulmonary disease (COPD)

Anesthesia for Ear, Nose, and Throat and Oral Surgery

Answers and Discussion

The authors have made every effort to thoroughly verify the answers to the questions that appear on the preceding pages. As in any text, however, some inaccuracies and ambiguities may occur. If in doubt, please consult the indicated reference. When no page number(s) are cited, the reference is to a journal article or to a refresher course lecture that should be read in its entirety.

The Editors

230. (B) Isolated palsy of the cricothyroids is extremely rare but can occur if the superior laryngeal nerve is damaged during thyroidectomy when the superior thyroid artery is being tied. Temporary paralysis of this muscle can occur following local anesthesia of the throat and larynx leading to a "gruff" voice. (**Ref. 36,** pp. 1020–1023)

231. (D) The interarytenoid (transverse arytenoid) is an unpaired muscle, inserting on the posterior surface of each arytenoid cartilage. The oblique arytenoids are thin bands that cross posteriorly in the midline and run from the muscular process of the arytenoid to the aryepiglottic fold and blend into the aryepiglottic muscle.

These arytenoid muscles appose the vocal cords when they contract. (**Ref. 18,** pp. 1255–1256)

232. **(D)** The extrinsic muscles move the larynx as a unit, whereas the intrinsic muscles move the different individual components located within the larynx. The main function of the extrinsic muscles is to depress and to elevate the larynx during deglutition. The principal depressor muscles of the larynx are the sternothyroid, the sternohyoid, and the omohyoid muscles. (**Ref. 18,** pp. 584–585)

233. **(B)** The mandibular branch of the trigeminal nerve supplies the sensation of touch to the anterior two-thirds of the tongue through the lingual nerve. The taste sensation is carried by the chorda tympani nerve, which is a branch of the facial nerve. (**Ref. 18,** pp. 1322–1323)

234. **(C)** Airway protection involves elevation and closure of the larynx during swallowing. Elevation is achieved by contraction of the strap muscles. Closure involves three sphincters: the epiglottic and aryepiglottic folds (which play only a minor role), the false vocal folds, and the true vocal folds. (**Ref. 18,** pp. 1328–1330)

235. **(C)** The reason for this is that the abductor muscles receive a greater number of nerve fibers than do the adductors, and they are therefore more vulnerable. When there is a pure abductor palsy on one side, both cords meet in the midline during phonation, because the adductors are intact. On inspiration, however, the cord on the affected side remains fixed in the midline, and the cord on the intact side moves to a position of full abduction. (**Ref. 40,** pp. 478–479)

236. **(C)** A hematoma in the neck that compromises the airway is a major emergency requiring immediate intervention. The hematoma must be opened at the bedside and must be evacuated without general anesthesia. Once the airway is reestablished, the patient can be safely taken back to the operating room to explore the wound for surgical hemostasis. (**Ref. 25,** pp. 339–347)

237. **(A)** It is important to appreciate the likelihood of fires during laser surgery and to take all necessary precautions to prevent such

a potentially disastrous complication. The minimum amount of oxygen that is consistent with acceptable peripheral oxygen saturation should be used. Nitrous oxide, which also supports combustion, should be avoided. Oxygen can and should be mixed with nonflammable gases, such as air, nitrogen, or helium. An FiO_2 of 0.6 to 0.8 should be perfectly acceptable in all but the exceptional patient. The management of endotracheal fires requires immediate discontinuation of oxygen, removal of the burning endotracheal tube, and reintubation of the trachea. Rigid bronchoscopy should be performed to check for and remove debris. Mask ventilation is almost certainly doomed to failure, in view of the thermal response in the upper and lower airway. (**Ref. 32,** p. 2017)

238. **(D)** Injury to tissues during laser surgery ensues when scattered or deflected laser beams come into direct contact with unprotected tissue. Stray carbon dioxide laser can cause corneal damage and NYD Yag laser beams can damage pigmented structures, such as the retina. Protective goggles must be worn by all personnel in the operating room and the patient's eyes must be protected with wet eye patches. Fetal abnormalities in pregnant women are clearly not a possible complication of ENT laser surgery, since there is no way in which even the most wayward laser beam could come into direct contact with fetal tissues. (**Ref. 32,** pp. 2016–2017)

239. **(D)** Some of the precautions that can be taken are using a metal ET tube, jet ventilation without using an ET tube, and using the lowest possible concentration of oxygen during ventilation. Laser surgery in itself is prone to promote fires. Both oxygen and nitrous oxide support combustion. Thus, such a mixture is undesirable in laser surgery in the pharynx or larynx. (**Ref. 32,** pp. 2016–2017)

240. **(B)** Under these conditions, the wires must be cut immediately and the patient must be intubated orally. Wire cutters must be at the bedside both in the recovery room and in the patient's room. Mask resuscitation may not succeed in the presence of blood, secretions, or vomitus in the oropharynx. The tongue may also obstruct the oropharynx, making mask ventilation very difficult or impossible. Mask ventilation must be used only while waiting for

wire cutters, or if oral intubation was unsuccessful and a tracheostomy is being performed. Nasal fiberoptic intubation is not an option under these emergency conditions. (**Ref. 7,** p. 1533)

241. (**B**)   It is wise to avoid sedation in the patients who obstruct their airway when they fall asleep. For this reason, it is recommended that narcotics be avoided in these patients. If sedation cannot be avoided, a small dose of a benzodiazepine should be used. These patients must be monitored very carefully, both in the operating room and, particularly, during the recovery period. Endotracheal intubation and securing the airway are extremely important. The visualization of the additus may be difficult because of redundant soft tissues, and this will lead to difficulties in intubating the trachea. (**Ref. 36,** pp. 426–427)

242. (**A**)   The Klippel–Feil syndrome is associated with a short neck as the result of fusion of cervical vertebrae, low hairline, and often an elevation of the scapula, known as the Sprengel's deformity. Tracheal intubation may be difficult or impossible by the conventional methods. Short extremities are not associated with Klippel–Feil syndrome. (**Ref. 26,** p. 582)

243. (**C**)   Halothane increases the sensitivity of the myocardium to the catecholamines, and the cause of the arrhythmias is believed to be the reentry mechanism. The incidence of arrhythmias from pancuronium increases during halothane anesthesia. Pancuronium causes an increase in the heart rate and blood pressure because of its vagolytic action and also by increasing the circulating catecholamine and norepinephrine. Increased production and decreased neuronal reuptake of norepinephrine has been suggested as a possible side effect of pancuronium. (**Ref. 32,** pp. 409, 1108)

244. (**A**)   Tracheotomy is usually free of major complications, but it is by no means an entirely benign procedure. The immediate complications include damage to the recurrent laryngeal nerve, minor hemorrhage, and the creation of a false passage or of a tracheoesophageal fistula. Late complications include massive hemorrhage from an exposed and eroded innominate artery and tracheal stenosis at or below the level of the tracheal stoma. Massive air embolization is extremely unlikely, unless the tracheotomy is performed as part of a radical neck dissection or other major craniofacial procedure. Minor complications include aspiration of blood during the performance of the tracheotomy and low-grade infection of the surgical site. Pneumothorax and subcutaneous emphysema are also possible sequelae of a hastily performed tracheotomy. (**Ref. 7,** p. 1121)

245. **(C)** A number of morbidly obese patients are hypoxic and hypercarbic because of increased oxygen consumption and increased carbon dioxide production. Heavy or sometimes even light sedation can push them over the edge, leading to hypoxemia. Transtracheal injection of epinephrine is of no use since the tracheal mucosa is not very vascular. (**Ref. 40,** pp. 541–542)

246. **(A)** Temporomandibular joint arthritis, along with cervical and cricoarytenoid arthritis, can make intubation very difficult or even impossible. There is an increased incidence of ischemic heart disease in these patients, presumably secondary to corticosteroid therapy. Obstructive lung disease is not usually associated with rheumatoid arthritis. (**Ref. 40,** pp. 635–636)

247. **(E)** Danazol is an androgen derivative that increases the plasma C_1 inhibitor. Prophylaxis with danazol should be initiated at least 10 days prior to the surgery. Fresh frozen plasma is a natural source of C_1 inhibitor. It should be administered at least 40 minutes prior to surgery. (**Ref. 40,** pp. 712–713)

248. **(C)** The combined use of epinephrine and cocaine contributed to the occurrence of cardiac arrhythmias. Cocaine inhibits the neuronal reuptake of catecholamines, and this leads to their increased concentration at the receptor site. In conjunction with exogenously administered epinephrine, cocaine can cause fatal arrhythmias unless the dose of both drugs is strictly limited. (**Ref. 26,** pp. 868–871)

249. **(A)** Bacteremia reflects the entrance of the normal upper airway bacterial flora into the circulation, secondary to trauma. Epistaxis may follow mucosal injury, and this can be minimized by proper shrinking of the mucosa using cocaine or neosynephrine. Sore throat is a side effect of tracheal intubation whether it is done nasally or orally. (**Ref. 32,** p. 537)

142 / 9: Anesthesia for ENT and Oral Surgery

250. **(A)** PEEP is not helpful in laryngeal edema. Racemic epinephrine, administered in a dose of 0.05 mL/kg in 2 mL of saline and IV Decadron 0.1 to 0.2 mg/kg are useful in decreasing the swelling. Assisted ventilation may be needed temporarily if the edema is causing partial obstruction. (**Ref. 40,** p. 854)

251. **(B)** In children the larynx is situated more cephalad (C_4) and anterior when compared to the adult larynx. A child's epiglottis is stiffer and narrower than the adult counterpart, and lifting the epiglottis using a straight blade is recommended for intubation. The narrowest part of the child's airway is at the level of the cricoid cartilage. This mandates that a minimal leak technique be used for intubation. A tight seal can lead to circumferential edema below the level of the cords, resulting in an upper airway obstruction following extubation. (**Ref. 36,** pp. 2161–2163)

252. **(C)** Since the oxygen reserve is a function of the FRC, the obese patient with considerably lower FRC than the normal person, will desaturate much faster. In a baby, the reserve may be comparable to a normal-sized adult kg for kg but the oxygen requirement is doubled and this leads to faster desaturation. (**Ref. 32,** pp. 1758–1759; **Ref 41,** p. 542)

253. **(A)** Acromegaly is the disorder associated with excessive secretion of growth hormone by an eosinophilic adenoma of the anterior pituitary. There is skeletal as well as soft tissue overgrowth leading to all the problems mentioned. (**Ref. 41,** pp. 510–511)

254. **(B)** If the mass is large, the airway is kept patent by the chest wall tone and the force of inspiration. Administering muscle relaxants can jeopardize this. Debulking the tumor prior to surgery, or intubating the patient without relaxants to maintain spontaneous respiration until the tumor is resected, is relatively safe. (**Ref. 24,** pp. 398–399)

255. **(B)** Failed or difficult endotracheal intubation is the most common cause of anesthetic-induced maternal mortality. In the absence of fetal distress, do not continue the procedure without securing the airway with an ET tube. Nondepolarizing relaxants should not be administered to a parturient who is difficult to intubate. Awakening the patient and offering an epidural is a viable

option. Small incremental doses of the local anesthetic should be administered in the epidural catheter to avoid intravascular injection and any subsequent complication that may necessitate tracheal intubation. (**Ref. 36,** p. 2084)

256. (B) Cricoarytenoid arthritis is common and is manifested by pain on phonation, hoarseness, odynophagia, and sometimes a sense of fullness in the oropharynx. Synovial destruction and vertebral erosion along with ligamentous changes may lead to cervical spine instability. Atlantoaxial instability may lead to subluxation and cord compression. Micrognathia and COPD are not seen in rheumatoid arthritis as part of the disease process. (**Ref. 40,** p. 633)

10

Anesthesia for Plastic and Reconstructive Surgery

DIRECTIONS (Questions 257–261): Each of the questions or incomplete statements below is followed by five suggested answers or completions. Select the **one** that is best in each case.

257. The anesthesia technique of choice for finger reimplantation is
   A. general anesthesia with deliberate hypotension
   B. local anesthesia
   C. axillary block
   D. Bier block
   E. balanced, light general anesthesia

258. A pneumatic tourniquet on the lower extremity can be left inflated safely for
   A. 30 minutes
   B. 60 minutes
   C. 90 minutes
   D. 120 minutes
   E. 150 minutes

259. If a vasopressor must be used during a transverse rectus abdominis musculocutaneous flap (TRAM) procedure, the agent of choice is
   A. dopamine
   B. ephedrine
   C. epinephrine
   D. phenylephrine
   E. norepinephrine

260. Which of the following is true about patients with extensive thermal injury?
   A. succinylcholine can be used safely
   B. they are resistant to nondepolarising muscle relaxants
   C. the selection of the proper anesthetic agent is critical
   D. these patients are severely hypermetabolic
   E. serum catecholamine levels are decreased

261. After a massive third-degree burn, fluid replacement during the first 24 hours should be
   A. 1.0 mL/kg/% of burn
   B. 2.0 mL/kg/% of burn
   C. 4.0 mL/kg/% of burn
   D. 0.1 mL/kg/% of burn
   E. 10 mL/kg/% of burn

DIRECTIONS (Questions 262–266): For each of the questions or incomplete answers below, **one** or **more** of the answers or completions are correct. Select
   A. if only 1, 2, and 3 are correct
   B. if only 1 and 3 are correct
   C. if only 2 and 4 are correct
   D. if only 4 is correct
   E. if all are correct

---

262. In anesthesia for a free muscle transfer procedure, which of the following may seriously affect the success of the operation?
   1. hypotension
   2. hypothermia
   3. hypovolemia
   4. infusion of low molecular weight dextran

10: Anesthesia for Plastic and Reconstructive Surgery

263. The clinical response to extensive burns includes
  1. myocardial depression
  2. hypovolemia
  3. glucose intolerance
  4. hypoproteinemia

264. The primary pulmonary pathogenesis of inhalation injury includes
  1. carbon monoxide poisoning
  2. direct thermal injury to the airway
  3. decrease in surfactant
  4. inhalation of the products of combustion

265. When intravenous regional anesthesia is used
  1. a double cuff is not necessary if the procedure lasts less than 45 minutes
  2. epinephrine should be added to the local anesthetic solution
  3. when bupivacaine is used, anesthesia is maintained after the tourniquet is released
  4. systemic anesthetic toxicity is a potential problem

266. In case of severe facial trauma
  1. an esophageal obturator should be used
  2. blind nasal intubation may be indicated
  3. tracheostomy is the technique of choice
  4. fiberoptic intubation may be the best approach

Anesthesia for Plastic and Reconstructive Surgery

Answers and Discussion

The authors have made every effort to thoroughly verify the answers to the questions that appear on the preceding pages. As in any text, however, some inaccuracies and ambiguities may occur. If in doubt, please consult the indicated reference. When no page number(s) are cited, the reference is to a journal article or to a refresher course lecture that should be read in its entirety.

The Editors

257. (C) There is some controversy on this subject. The reference textbook strongly recommends an axillary block with bupivacaine (0.5%) with epinephrine with the expectation that the block will last 12 to 16 hours. The sedation recommended is diazepam and pentobarbital. Today few anesthesiologists would agree with this approach and would probably favor a light general anesthetic. The reason for this is obvious when we consider that reimplantation may take considerably longer than 12 to 16 hours and, further, that even well-sedated patients become restless when lying on an uncomfortable operating table hour after hour. (**Ref. 16,** p. 1088)

148 / 10: Anesthesia for Plastic and Reconstructive Surgery

258. **(D)** The tourniquet must be released after a maximum inflation time of 120 minutes. It can be reinflated again after an interval of 20 minutes, provided that there is adequate blood flow during the 20 minutes of down time. (**Ref. 16,** pp. 1096–1097)

259. **(A)** Vasopressors should be avoided entirely if at all possible, and hypotension should be corrected by administering additional intravenous fluid and by lightening the general anesthesia. If this approach is unsatisfactory and a vasopressor must be used to avoid cardiovascular collapse, dopamine in small doses (5 µg/kg/min) is the drug of choice. Use of any of the other vasopressors may well doom the surgical procedure to failure. (**Ref. 16,** p. 1032 and the author's experience)

260. **(D)** Patients with severe burns become hypermetabolic a few hours after the injury and remain so almost until they are completely recovered. They will be hyperthermic, tachycardic, and tachypneic. They will have increased catabolism and increased circulating catecholamine levels. This must be taken into consideration when nutritional and ventilatory needs are under review. Ventilation must be sufficient to cope with the markedly increased carbon dioxide production, and nutrition must try to satisfy the huge caloric expenditure. Because of the hypermetabolic state, the burned patient is particularly prone to hypothermia during anesthesia and must be protected by raising the temperature in the operating room and by warming all the IV fluids. (**Ref. 7,** pp. 1421–1422)

261. **(A)** This is the so-called Parkland formula for adults. It calls for 4 mL/kg/% burn lactated Ringer's solution during the first 24 hours. Fifty percent of the calculated dose should be given during the first 8 hours and the remaining 50% during the next 16 hours. It is a reasonable guideline but is no more than that. Once vigorous fluid replacement therapy has begun, the best determinants for the adequacy of fluid replacement are urine output, urine specific gravity, and heart rate. Blood pressure is not a reliable guide in view of the very high level of circulating catecholamines. In extensively burned patients, particularly in the elderly, it may be necessary to monitor cardiovascular stability with a pulmonary artery catheter. (**Ref. 16,** p. 685)

262. **(A)** The success of this type of surgery is contingent upon the patency and fullness of the microscopically anastomosed vessels. Hypovolemia and hypothermia both lead to vascular spasm by themselves. Attempting to correct the resulting hypotension with peripherally acting vasopressors makes a bad situation very much worse and is very likely to lead to the loss of the pedicle or free graft. It is critical that these patients be kept euvolemic and warm. Any decrease in blood pressure due to blood loss or depth of anesthesia must be corrected by generous replacement therapy and reestablishing a light level of anesthesia. (**Ref. 16,** pp. 1032–1035)

263. **(E)** All of these are characteristic clinical responses to massive thermal injuries. The reason for the myocardial depression has never been fully substantiated although the appearance of a myocardial depressor factor has been postulated. Hypovolemia is due to massive extravasation and loss of intravascular volume into the tissues in and around the affected areas. The glucose intolerance is present in the early phases only and is due to the massive increase in the circulating catecholamines. The protein loss is greatest 8 to 12 hours after the injury, and this in turn will aggravate the already existing tissue edema. (**Ref. 16,** pp. 684–685)

264. **(C)** The most significant pathogenic factor is the inhalation of the products of combustion. Smoke, particularly from plastics and other synthetic substances, produces severe injury to the lower respiratory tract and is primarily responsible for the development of the clinical picture of ARDS. Carbon monoxide causes little, if any, direct pulmonary pathology. Its affinity for hemoglobin produces systemic effects that may be fatal but are not primarily pulmonary. The direct thermal injury is usually limited to the upper airway. The exception to this rule is the injury produced by superheated steam, which may indeed cause parenchymal thermal injury. The decrease of surfactant is a secondary manifestation and is part of the ARDS complex. Prompt endotracheal intubation is mandatory in suspected airway thermal injury. Delay may make intubation extremely difficult or impossible and will require emergency tracheostomy under very unfavorable conditions. (**Ref. 16,** pp. 688–690)

265. (D) There is a real risk of systemic local anesthetic toxicity if the tourniquet is accidentally released early. It can be safely deflated after 40 minutes. Between 20 and 40 minutes, the tourniquet may be deflated and rapidly reinflated several times. A double cuff is recommended, since tourniquet pain may appear in less than 45 minutes. A double tourniquet somewhat increases the risk of local anesthetic leakage and is also more likely to be deflated accidentally. Epinephrine should not be added to the local anesthetic solution. It is not only totally unnecessary but may cause systemic complications when the tourniquet is released. The anesthesia dissipates very rapidly after release of the tourniquet, and the use of bupivacaine does not appreciably prolong it. (**Ref. 7,** pp. 856–857)

266. (D) Obviously the approach to airway management is largely dependent upon the type and extent of the facial injuries and the possibility of concomitant cranial and/or cervical injuries. Establishment of a reliable airway is critical. A tracheostomy may be required but is hardly ever the technique of choice. Fiberoptic oral intubation is probably the technique of choice in many situations, since it permits a direct and relatively nontraumatic approach to the glottis and beyond. In cases of suspected tracheolaryngeal injury it is almost mandatory. Blind nasal intubation, although impressive to the uninitiated bystander, is contraindicated, since in fresh and severe facial trauma the possibility of cribriform plate fracture cannot be ruled out readily. There are cases on record where blind nasotracheal intubation became blind (and potentially blinding) nasocranial intubation. The esophageal obturator should not be used. Its use is fraught with danger and it offers minimal, if any, benefits. (**Ref. 7, p.** 1418)

11
Anesthesia for Thoracic Surgery

DIRECTIONS (Questions 267–272): Each of the questions or incomplete statements below is followed by five suggested answers or completions. Select the **one** that is best in each case.

267. Resectional pulmonary surgery is probably contraindicated if
   A. resting PaO_2 on room air is 88 mm Hg
   B. resting $PaCO_2$ is 52 mm Hg
   C. FEV_1 is 80% of predicted
   D. MVV is less than 75% of predicted
   E. patient is dyspneic after climbing three flights of stairs

268. Vigorous head movement may shift the tip of the endotracheal tube
   A. not at all when properly secured
   B. 1 to 2 cm
   C. 2 to 3 cm
   D. 4 to 5 cm
   E. more than 5 cm

269. In the anesthetized paralyzed patient in the lateral decubitus position, with the chest open
   A. the dependent lung receives relatively less perfusion
   B. the nondependent lung receives relatively more perfusion
   C. the dependent lung remains relatively poorly ventilated
   D. the nondependent lung will be hyperventilated
   E. both lungs will be better ventilated

270. In monitoring during one-lung anesthesia, all these modalities must be used EXCEPT
   A. pulse oximeter
   B. cuff blood pressure
   C. ECG
   D. capnography
   E. arterial cannula

271. Which of the following is NOT an indication for fiberoptic bronchoscopy?
   A. vertebral artery insufficiency
   B. removal of fragile foreign body
   C. poor dental status
   D. increased patient comfort
   E. ability to enter smaller bronchi

272. Airway resistance increase caused by histamine release is LEAST likely following
   A. thiopental
   B. thiamylal
   C. fentanyl
   D. morphine
   E. meperidine

DIRECTIONS (Questions 273–286): For each of the questions or incomplete answers below, **one** or **more** of the answers or completions are correct. Select

- **A.** if only 1, 2, and 3 are correct
- **B.** if only 1 and 3 are correct
- **C.** if only 2 and 4 are correct
- **D.** if only 4 is correct
- **E.** if all are correct

273. In a patient with AIDS, thoracoscopic pulmonary biopsy may be extremely difficult because of
   1. oral candidiasis
   2. pneumocystis pneumonia
   3. Kaposi's sarcoma
   4. hypertrophic tonsils and adenoids

274. The absolute indications for one-lung anesthesia include
   1. bronchial sleeve resection
   2. control of spillage from the nondependent lung
   3. bronchopleural fistula
   4. surgical convenience

275. The complications of mediastinoscopy include
   1. innominate artery injury and hemorrhage
   2. pneumothorax
   3. esophageal perforation
   4. vocal cord paralysis

276. The major goals of premedication prior to thoracic surgery are
   1. decreasing the incidence of emergence delirium
   2. anxiety relief
   3. decreasing the incidence of nausea and vomiting
   4. amnesia

277. Arterial oxygenation under one-lung anesthesia can be enhanced by
   1. PEEP to the dependent lung
   2. PEEP to the nondependent lung
   3. CPAP to the nondependent lung
   4. CPAP to the dependent lung

278. The blood flow to the dependent lung is increased during one-lung ventilation by
    1. hypoxic pulmonary vasoconstriction
    2. reducing lung volume
    3. gravity
    4. absorption atelectasis

279. PaO_2 will NOT be increased during one-lung ventilation by
    1. increased tidal volumes
    2. intermittent manual hyperventilation
    3. changing I–E ratios
    4. PEEP

280. Fiberoptic confirmation of correct double-lumen tube placement is required
    1. in all cases
    2. in very obese patients
    3. with all left-sided tubes
    4. with all right-sided tubes

281. Iatrogenic perforation of the esophagus is usually due to
    1. gastrointestinal endoscopy
    2. traumatic endotracheal intubation
    3. bougineage
    4. nasogastric tube

282. In patients undergoing thymectomy for myasthenia gravis, monitoring should routinely include
    1. central venous pressure line
    2. mechanomyography
    3. Swan–Ganz catheter
    4. pulse oximetry

283. The indications for bronchopulmonary lavage include
    1. alveolar proteinosis
    2. inhalation of radioactive dust
    3. cystic fibrosis
    4. bronchiectasis

284. Preparation of a patient with COPD for thoracic surgery should include
1. cessation of smoking
2. steroids
3. chest physiotherapy
4. beta agonists

285. Epidural analgesia for post-thoracotomy pain
1. should be established preoperatively
2. should combine local anesthetics and opioids
3. significantly reduces postoperative complications
4. is superior to other forms of analgesia

286. In anesthesia for single-lung transplant
1. extracorporeal bypass is required
2. a pulmonary artery catheter is required
3. a double-lumen tube is required
4. right heart failure is a major intraoperative problem

Anesthesia for Thoracic Surgery

Answers and Discussion

The authors have made every effort to thoroughly verify the answers to the questions that appear on the preceding pages. As in any text, however, some inaccuracies and ambiguities may occur. If in doubt, please consult the indicated reference. When no page number(s) are cited, the reference is to a journal article or to a refresher course lecture that should be read in its entirety.

The Editors

267. **(B)** When a patient retains carbon dioxide, it is an indication of significant respiratory failure and carries a grave prognostic meaning. If it can be shown that this degree of hypercarbia is accompanied by a marked decrease in FEV_1 to levels of 800 to 1000 mL, the likelihood of serious postoperative problems approaches 100%. Under these conditions, the thoracotomy alone, even without any pulmonary resection, may lead to long-term and even permanent ventilatory support. Morbidity and mortality are extremely high in these patients. (**Ref. 24,** p. 15)

268. **(D)** Radiologic studies have documented that vigorous flexion and extension of the head may move the tip of the endotracheal

tube as much as 4 to 5 cm. The implications of this observation are obvious. Ideally, the tube should be placed so that with the head in the neutral position, the tip of the tube is about 5 cm above the carina. Since the adult trachea is 10 to 12 cm long, this will allow the tube to move 2 to 2.5 cm in either direction without causing problems. Radiographic findings of less than 3 cm from the carina to the tip of the endotracheal tube should be viewed with suspicion. If the radiograph was taken with the patient's head in extension, subsequent flexion of the head may advance the tip of the tube into the right main-stem bronchus. (**Ref. 24,** p. 65)

269. (C) Opening the chest wall significantly affects the relative ventilation and perfusion of the dependent (lower) and nondependent (upper) lung. The dependent lung will continue to receive greater perfusion and less ventilation. The nondependent lung will not have any increased circulation but will be relatively hyperventilated because the chest wall no longer contributes to compliance. In the paralyzed patient, at least theoretically, the mismatch is made worse because the diaphragm in the dependent area is displaced much less than in the nondependent area.

When surgical retractors or packs restrict the motion of the nondependent lung, the situation will be improved and more ventilation will be directed toward the dependent lung. Since this lung already receives more perfusion, the ventilation–perfusion ratio will be improved. (**Ref. 24,** pp. 201–202)

270. (E) During one-lung anesthesia, there will always be a significant shunt. It is therefore essential to monitor arterial oxygenation. Some authorities still recommend that an arterial cannula be placed in every patient who will undergo one-lung anesthesia. Actually, there is no need for invasive monitoring; pulse oximetry is a perfectly satisfactory method of monitoring these patients. There is ample experimental evidence that pulse oximetry correlates sufficiently well with arterial oxygen tension measurements. Unless the patient has some other indication for an arterial line, this admittedly benign, but nevertheless invasive monitoring technique may safely be omitted. (**Ref. 24,** pp. 311–312)

271. (B) Fiberoptic bronchoscopy has many advantages. It is much less uncomfortable than rigid bronchoscopy. It can be performed in patients who cannot extend their neck or who have fragile upper teeth. Two additional major advantages of fiberoptic bronchoscopy are that much more distal bronchi can be inspected and biopsied, and that closed-circuit television imaging has become a valuable tool in teaching and in documenting pathology. Its sole major disadvantage is that it is not suitable for the removal of highly friable foreign bodies or for suction removal of large amounts of blood or inspissated secretions. (**Ref. 24,** p. 325)

272. **(C)** Both thiopental and thiamylal produce the release of histamine. The only barbiturate induction agent that does not produce histamine is methohexital. Among the narcotics, morphine and meperidine cause histamine release; fentanyl, sufentanyl, and alfentanyl do not. Etomidate rarely causes histamine release, and ketamine actually has bronchodilator effects. The histamine release caused by morphine and meperidine cannot be antagonized by naloxone. Of the nondepolarizing muscle relaxants, only vecuronium and pancuronium do not cause histamine release. The inhalation agents are bronchodilators and, on general principles, isoflurane seems to be the most satisfactory. (**Ref. 24,** pp. 349–350)

273. **(E)** Patients with clinical evidence of AIDS are very poor candidates for thoracic surgery. Thoracoscopic surgery requires one-lung anesthesia, which the AIDS patient may not be able to tolerate. Intubation with a double-lumen tube may be impossible because of oral candidiasis. In severe cases this may distort and obstruct the upper airway of the patient, and intubation even with a single-lumen tube may be extremely difficult or impossible, using the usual technique. Awake, fiberoptic intubation may be necessary. *P. carinii* infections produce copious, tenacious secretions, making ventilation difficult. Kaposi's sarcoma is an aggressive neoplasm in these patients and does not uncommonly appear in the upper airway. If a lung biopsy, or any other intrathoracic surgical procedure must be performed in an AIDS patient, a single-lumen endotracheal tube and two-lung ventilation is probably required. (**Ref. 24,** pp. 107–108)

274. **(A)** One-lung anesthesia is essential in a number of conditions. These include bronchial sleeve resection, accumulations of blood, pus, or debris in the nondependent lung (bronchiectasis, lung abscess, necrotic tissue, etc.), bronchopleural fistula, bronchopul-

monary lavage, single-lung transplant, and thoracoscopy. A "quiet lung" makes resectional surgery easier and faster, but it is not an absolute requirement. In certain patients, one-lung anesthesia may be technically very difficult. Some patients with extensive bilateral disease will not tolerate one-lung anesthesia. Under no circumstances should surgical convenience outweigh considerations of patient safety. The quiet lung should be made available whenever appropriate, since surgical dispatch is generally to the patient's benefit. (**Ref. 24,** pp. 371-372)

275. (E) All of these are possible complications of mediastinoscopy. If the mediastinal mass is large, the airway may already be compromised, and both intraoperative and postoperative problems must be anticipated. Pneumothorax is a real possibility. Therefore, nitrous oxide is best avoided, and a postoperative chest x-ray must be obtained. Not uncommonly, the mediastinal mass is a thymoma, and hence the possibility of a subclinical myasthenia gravis must be a consideration. The patient must be observed very closely in the immediate postoperative period, because the formation of a mediastinal hematoma or vocal cord paralysis, secondary to recurrent laryngeal nerve injury, may lead to a rapid and rapidly disastrous upper airway obstruction. (**Ref. 24,** pp. 339-340)

276. (C) Anxiety relief is probably the most important consideration in premedication. Amnesia, analgesia, antisialagogue effects, achlorhydria, and hypnosis are also major goals. Anxiety relief is best accomplished by oral diazepam or parenteral lorazepam or midazolam. Morphine, meperidine, the barbiturates, and droperidol have many undesirable side effects and are best avoided. Preoperative pain is rarely a problem in these patients. Hence, analgesia is not required. Narcotics may of course be given just prior to induction, but such use comes properly under the heading of anesthesia rather than premedication. Achlorhydria is indicated in only those patients in whom reflux has been a real problem. Antisialagogues were used routinely in the past. Current thinking limits their use to patients who are likely to have multiple oropharyngeal manipulations. Emergence delirium and postoperative nausea and vomiting have a low enough incidence to make routine pharmacologic preventive measures both medically and economically unsound. (**Ref. 24,** pp. 258-261)

160 / 11: Anesthesia for Thoracic Surgery

277. **(B)** Unless there is considerable bilateral pulmonary disease, patients will tolerate one-lung anesthesia well and will maintain good arterial oxygen levels, provided the FiO_2 is maintained at 80% to 100%. If the oxygen saturation decreases, the first step is to check the position and patency of the double-lumen tube. Assuming that the tube is in the correct position and that the need for one-lung ventilation still exists, the next step should be to add 5 to 10 cm H_2O PEEP to the dependent lung. If this is still not sufficient to increase the oxygen saturation to satisfactory levels, 5 to 10 cm H_2O CPAP can be added to the nondependent lung. PEEP and CPAP should be adjusted until satisfactory oxygenation is achieved. An occasional patient will be hypoxemic on one-lung ventilation, regardless of what PEEP or CPAP is used. These patients must be returned to two-lung ventilation, at least temporarily, without any undue delay. (**Ref. 24,** pp. 216–217)

278. **(B)** The primary reasons for increased blood flow to the dependent lung during one-lung anesthesia are gravity and pulmonary hypoxic vasoconstriction (HPV). The passive, gravity-dependent increase in blood flow is purely positional. The lower portions of the lung are always better perfused, and at the same time, they are less well ventilated. The HPV is a regulatory reflex that causes pulmonary vascular constriction in those areas that are poorly ventilated and hence relatively hypoxic. Thus, the area where blood is shunted from right to left (i.e., the entire nondependent lung during one-lung ventilation) will be vasoconstricted. This will markedly increase blood flow to the dependent lung, decrease the amount of shunted blood, and improve arterial oxygenation. The reduced lung volume in the dependent lung, as a result of pressure from the viscera and the awkward positioning, will reduce blood flow to this lung and so will absorption atelectasis that may take place in some areas of the dependent lung. (**Ref. 24,** p. 211)

279. **(A)** Contrary to popular belief, increasing the tidal volume of ventilation, intermittent manual hyperventilation of the dependent lung, or adjusting the E–I ratios in various ways did not increase PaO_2 in the patients during one-lung ventilation. PEEP does improve PaO_2 in many patients but is a mixed blessing. It not only increases residual functional capacity of the dependent lung, but it also increases the vascular resistance in this area and hence has a

negative effect on arterial oxygenation. The cautious use of PEEP will favor the positive effect, particularly in those patients who had a "bad" lung to begin with. If the dependent lung was normal prior to the institution of one-lung ventilation, the chances are that PEEP will either produce no effect on arterial oxygenation or will actually decrease it. (**Ref. 24,** pp. 212–214)

280. **(D)** Studies have shown that a significant percentage of the currently used PVC double-lumen tubes were incorrectly placed. The traditional methods of checking correct placement (i.e., auscultation and inspection) are usually satisfactory to confirm accurate placement of a left-sided tube. These techniques are unreliable when checking the position of a right-sided tube, since partial or complete occlusion of the right upper-lobe bronchus may go undetected by physical examination. In many patients with good lungs, this probably makes little difference, since these patients will do well when only the right middle and lower lobes are ventilated. Yet, to avoid right upper-lobe atelectasis in good lungs or severe hypoxemia in inpatients with generalized pulmonary disease, the position of the right double-lumen tube must be checked with the fiberoptic bronchoscope. This check should be performed both after induction and again, after the patient has been turned into the lateral decubitus position. (**Ref. 24,** pp. 384–387)

281. **(A)** All of these are known to cause esophageal perforation with ensuing mediastinitis unless promptly diagnosed and treated. The most common iatrogenic cause of esophageal perforation is esophagogastric endoscopy. The use of bougies for esophageal dilatation is also a common cause of this potentially fatal iatrogenic complication. Traumatic endotracheal or inadvertent esophageal intubation have caused perforation. In the latter cases the perforation is usually at the level of the cricopharyngeus muscle, whereas the endoscope usually causes a perforation in the distal segment. The bougie causes the perforation wherever the stricture is. Nasogastric or orogastric suction has caused esophageal perforation in the neonate but would be extremely rare in the adult patient. (**Ref. 24,** p. 393)

282. **(D)** There is no justification for invasive monitoring in these patients unless there is a history of co-existing, significant cardiovascular disease. Pulse oximetry is standard. The newly intro-

duced, integrated EMG monitoring system and Accelograph acceleration monitor have been very helpful in following the train-of-four response and the recovery from even minute doses of nondepolarizing muscle relaxants. These instruments are capable of printing a hard copy of the findings, which may be very helpful in following the patient's recovery. They also make an excellent teaching tool. (**Ref. 24,** p. 405)

283. **(E)** Bronchopulmonary lavage is a heroic undertaking that has proven highly beneficial in otherwise unmanageable cases of alveolar proteinosis and cystic fibrosis. Inhalation of radioactive dust and bronchiectasis are also listed as indications, but they must be indeed rare applications. Anesthesia for bronchopulmonary lavage absolutely demands the use of a double-lumen endotracheal tube. Placement of this tube is critical, and the cuffs must be absolutely occlusive to prevent leakage of the large volume of irrigating fluid into the ventilated lung. The procedure is fraught with intraoperative and postoperative complications. (**Ref. 24,** pp. 435–437)

284. **(C)** Many patients scheduled for pulmonary surgery have at least some COPD by virtue of age, smoking, industrial exposure, etc. Since much of thoracic surgery is not of an emergency nature, there is usually time to improve the patient's pulmonary status. This is best accomplished with steroids and beta-2 agonists. The steroids should be given for several days prior to surgery, whereas the beta-2 agonists are best administered by inhalation just before the induction of anesthesia.

Acute smoking cessation probably has no benefits unless at least 8 weeks are available for a smoke-free period. The single prospective study showed that with less than 5 weeks of smoke-free time the patients had almost twice as many pulmonary complications as those who never stopped smoking. After 8 weeks the complication rate was less than that seen in the smokers. Chest physiotherapy is expensive and unrewarding except in a very few isolated cases. (**Ref. 5,** #224)

285. **(A)** Thoracic epidural analgesia is becoming a widely used method to manage the usually severe post-thoracotomy pain. There is accumulating evidence that the combination of local anesthetic and opioid permits earlier ambulation and respiratory

toilet, thus reducing the incidence of postoperative pulmonary complications. It may also shorten hospital stay. Ideally, it should be introduced preoperatively because thoracic epidural analgesia in an unconscious or uncooperative patient is a hazardous undertaking. There is no clear evidence that epidural analgesia holds any significant advantage over patient-controlled IV analgesia or over an interpleural block. (**Ref. 24,** pp. 571 et seq.)

286. **(C)** Both single- and double-lung transplants are becoming increasingly popular. In the young patient with end-stage pulmonary disease, it is the only form of therapy. Idiopathic pulmonary fibrosis is the most frequent but by no means sole indication. Extracorporeal bypass is usually required for double-lung transplants and is advocated by some groups for all single-lung transplants as well. It is not a requirement, however, and single-lung transplants can be done very satisfactorily without it. Although one-lung anesthesia is an obvious requirement even for the single-lung transplants, it need not be done with a double-lumen tube. According to the reference, a double-lumen tube is used mostly for right-lung transplants. Left-lung transplants are done with a Fogarty catheter placed under direct vision into the left main-stem bronchus. Right heart failure is the major hemodynamic problem, and this is the reason for requiring a central line. (**Ref. 24,** pp. 558–562)

12

Anesthesia for Cardiac Surgery

DIRECTIONS (Questions 287–297): Each of the questions or incomplete statements below is followed by five suggested answers or completions. Select the **one** that is best in each case.

287. Which of the following features of cardiovascular function do not change appreciably with aging?
  A. maximum heart rate
  B. cardiac output at rest
  C. early diastolic filling
  D. afterload
  E. resting heart rate

288. The most common cause of congestive heart failure in the elderly is
  A. coronary artery disease
  B. hypertension
  C. diastolic dysfunction
  D. systolic dysfunction
  E. idiopathic cardiomyopathy

289. The best evidence to support a perioperative myocardial infarction includes all of the following EXCEPT
    A. new Q waves on ECG
    B. tachycardia
    C. segmental wall motion abnormalities by 2-D echocardiography
    D. creatine kinase–MB fraction present
    E. troponin I present

290. The advantages of using intraoperative autologous cell savers include all the following EXCEPT
    A. removal of activated clotting factors
    B. short processing times
    C. low risk of air embolism
    D. lack of contamination
    E. removal of free hemoglobin and cellular debris

291. The most important factor determining the hematocrit after the initiation of cardiopulmonary bypass (CPB) is
    A. pre-CPB hematocrit
    B. red cell mass
    C. pre-CPB fluids
    D. pre-CPB renal function
    E. pump prime volume

292. Reducing the inflammatory response to cardiopulmonary bypass can be accomplished by
    A. aprotinin
    B. steroids
    C. high-dose opiates
    D. antihistamines
    E. prostaglandin inhibitors

293. Consistent decreases in the whole blood activated clotting time can be expected from
    A. hemodilution
    B. protamine
    C. aprotinin
    D. surgical incision
    E. hypothermia

294. Sites of temperature monitoring that, during rewarming, return to normal most rapidly and least rapidly, respectively, are which one of the following pairs?
   A. rectum and nasopharynx
   B. bladder and pulmonary artery
   C. arterial cannula and rectum
   D. myocardium and brain
   E. myocardium and nasopharynx

295. A 48-year-old female (50 kg, Hct 30%) presents with chronic mitral stenosis for mitral valve replacement. The pump prime volume is 2 L. 500 mL of IV fluids are given prior to CPB and urine output has been minimal. What most closely approximates the patient's estimated Hct after CPB is begun?
   A. 25%
   B. 21%
   C. 18%
   D. 15%
   E. 12%

296. A heart transplant recipient would be expected to have which of the following?
   A. hypertension and bradycardia from norepinephrine
   B. tachycardia from atropine
   C. tachycardia from pancuronium
   D. hypertension and bradycardia with phenylephrine
   E. tachycardia with norepinephrine

297. Which component of arterial blood pressure is most consistently reproducible by various techniques and under nonideal invasive monitoring conditions?
   A. dicrotic notch
   B. diastolic pressure
   C. pulse pressure
   D. mean pressure
   E. systolic pressure

DIRECTIONS (Questions 298–321): For each of the questions or incomplete answers below, **one** or **more** of the answers or completions are correct. Select
- **A.** if only 1, 2, and 3 are correct
- **B.** if only 1 and 3 are correct
- **C.** if only 2 and 4 are correct
- **D.** if only 4 is correct
- **E.** if all are correct

298. Which of the following statement(s) is (are) not correct?
1. retrograde cardioplegia can expose the right ventricle (RV) to inadequate protection
2. repeated doses of cardioplegia are necessary because of collateral flow
3. important components of myocardial protection are "cold, quiet, and empty"
4. cardioplegia is eucalcemic with respect to plasma

299. Important differences in pH stat and alpha stat blood gas management during cardiopulmonary bypass include
1. total CO_2 remains constant
2. net charge on proteins remains constant
3. CO_2 is added to the oxygenator
4. cerebral blood flow increases

300. The major mechanisms of myocardial injury during cardiac surgery include
1. chemical cardioplegia
2. antecedent ischemia
3. reperfusion injury
4. duration of the bypass

301. The use of "hot shot" cardioplegia has been shown to have the following advantages when given near the end of CPB
1. decreased rewarming time
2. improved post-ischemic metabolic recovery
3. reduced post-CPB atrial fibrillation
4. improved postoperative outcome

12: Anesthesia for Cardiac Surgery

302. The pharmacokinetic effects of hypothermic cardiopulmonary bypass include
    1. an initial drop in sufentanil concentration followed by gradual rise and peak at the termination of CPB
    2. sodium nitroprusside administration results in rapid release of CN⁻ and significant elevations of RBC thiocyanate
    3. volume of distribution of insulin and nitroglycerin are increased
    4. insignificant quantities of opioids are bound to oxygenators

303. The greatest potential hematological perturbation results from what features of cardiopulmonary bypass?
    1. exposure to non-endothelialized surfaces
    2. type of oxygenator
    3. release of thromboplastin
    4. hypothermia and hemodilution

304. The most common mechanisms of air embolism during cardiopulmonary bypass include
    1. improper removal of air from arterial line during flush maneuver
    2. inattention to venous reservoir level
    3. improper aortic cannulation site
    4. aortic root air during cardioplegia administration

305. The persistent popularity of nonpulsatile flow during cardiopulmonary bypass is attributable to which of the following?
    1. acceptable results from nonpulsatile perfusion
    2. increased cost and complexity of providing pulsatile perfusion
    3. no demonstrable superiority of nonpulsatile versus pulsatile perfusion
    4. lack of patentable pulsatile technology

306. Commercial sources of heparin for cardiopulmonary bypass include
    1. bovine lung tissue
    2. tissue mast cells
    3. porcine intestine
    4. monoclonal recombinant production

307. Heparin
   1. has an uncertain physiologic role
   2. unfractionated averages molecular weight of 50,000
   3. is most likely not a natural human agonist for antithrombin III
   4. has consistent potency per weight

308. Adequate anticoagulation for cardiopulmonary bypass is achieved when
   1. 300 U/kg heparin IV is administered
   2. heparin concentration of 3 U/mL whole blood
   3. ACT >300 sec
   4. aPTT >100 sec

309. Heparin resistance is associated with
   1. prior IV heparin therapy
   2. platelet count >700,000 or sepsis
   3. hypereosinophilic syndrome
   4. IV nitroglycerin therapy

310. Which of the following statement(s) about protamine is (are) NOT correct?
   1. it is a polycationic protein from salmon milt
   2. it has a single active site causing binding of heparin and anticoagulation
   3. it is a component of NPH insulin
   4. 10 mg will completely neutralize 1000 U of heparin

311. A 67-year-old male is anesthetized for CABG. He has been receiving IV heparin for treatment of unstable angina for 7 days. Baseline ACT is 110 sec and after a 400 µg/kg loading dose, his 5 min ACT stops at 300 sec. Which of the following are appropriate?
   1. stop the procedure; patient will die if placed on CPB
   2. administer additional heparin, 200 µg/kg, and recheck ACT
   3. check AT III level and give recombinant AT III
   4. administer 500 mL fresh frozen plasma

312. The protamine reactions can be characterized by
    1. hypotension
    2. anaphylaxis or a delayed anaphylactoid reaction
    3. pulmonary edema
    4. histamine release

313. The problems associated with the use of an intra-aortic balloon pump include
    1. ischemia
    2. embolization
    3. measurement of blood pressure
    4. dissection

314. The reasons myocardial function may be worse after CPB compared to before CPB include which of the following?
    1. prolonged aortic cross-clamp time
    2. ventriculostomy
    3. mitral valve replacement
    4. mitral valve repair

315. A 68-year-old male with insulin-dependent diabetes mellitus and severe CAD is weaned from CPB, AV paced at 97/min on dopamine 5 μg/kg/min. CO is 3.5 L/min with a pulmonary artery diastolic pressure (PAD) of 16. Protamine is started and 5 minutes later the MAP is 30 and the PAD is 40. The next steps are
    1. stop the protamine and administer epinephrine 100 μg IV bolus
    2. give heparin 300 μg/kg IV stat
    3. stop the protamine and administer norepinephrine 4 μg/min IV
    4. give PGE_1 0.1 μg/kg/min IV

316. The major mechanisms of action of antiarrhythmic drugs include the following:
    1. negative inotropy
    2. suppression of automaticity
    3. increased conduction velocity
    4. decreased conduction velocity

317. Patients also at risk for acute pulmonary hypertensive crises include which of the following?
   1. after mitral valve surgery in patients with preexisting pulmonary hypertension
   2. following emergent pulmonary embolectomy
   3. following heart transplantation
   4. heart surgery following vasectomy

318. The clinical uses for adenosine include
   1. treatment of re-entrant ventricular tachycardia
   2. termination of AV nodal re-entrant supraventricular tachycardia
   3. treatment of hypotension
   4. assessment of coronary flow reserve

319. Central venous pressure monitoring is useful for
   1. optimizing temporary pacing
   2. diagnosis of arrhythmias
   3. estimating RVEDP
   4. estimating LVEDV

320. Arterial pressure measurement differences from one location to another could be caused by
   1. atherosclerosis
   2. vasodilation
   3. resonance and filter frequency
   4. technique

321. The major limitations of intraoperative transesophageal echocardiography are
   1. anatomic incompatibility
   2. artifact interference
   3. lack of specificity
   4. detection of air

Anesthesia for Cardiac Surgery

Answers and Discussion

The authors have made every effort to thoroughly verify the answers to the questions that appear on the preceding pages. As in any text, however, some inaccuracies and ambiguities may occur. If in doubt, please consult the indicated reference. When no page number(s) are cited, the reference is to a journal article or to a refresher course lecture that should be read in its entirety.

The Editors

287. **(E)** Resting heart rate does not change and is relatively well preserved. Maximum heart rate, however, declines significantly, as does cardiac output both at rest and with exercise. The decrease in early diastolic filling is important physiologically because older patients become more dependent upon late diastolic filling (during atrial contraction) to augment end diastolic volume. This is in part a reflection of the decreased diastolic relaxation of the myocardium, which is an energy-dependent phenomenon. Afterload rises as the conductive vessels lose elasticity, and the cross-sectional area of the entire vascular bed diminishes. This results in a greater work load for the heart at a given flow. (**Ref. 23,** pp. 209–234)

Answers and Discussion: 287–290 / 173

288. **(C)** Although both coronary artery disease and hypertension are associated with the majority of patients who are elderly and have congestive heart failure, most of these patients have normal systolic function but have elevated LVEDP both at rest and during exercise. Markedly reduced diastolic function is characteristic. It reflects a stiff, noncompliant LV with slow filling, highly dependent upon atrial contraction. Diastole is an active, energy-requiring process, even more so than ventricular contraction. As such, diastole is more susceptible to ischemia and hypoxemia. Distinguishing systolic from diastolic dysfunction can be difficult, as both can coexist under some conditions. Determining which is causative is actually quite important because the appropriate therapeutic interventions are quite different (digitalis, nitrates, and diuretics for systolic dysfunction versus calcium channel blockers, beta blockers, ACE inhibitors, in the treatment of atrial fibrillation). Ischemic and valvular heart disease commonly have both systolic and diastolic dysfunction, and both must be treated simultaneously. (**Ref. 23,** pp. 209–234)

289. **(A)** New Q waves on a postoperative ECG are very good evidence of a very recent myocardial infarction. A tachycardia, while it may accompany ischemia and infarction, is not specific enough by itself to warrant diagnosis. New segmental wall motion abnormalities are useful but difficult to diagnose accurately in the clinical setting and are subject to changes in loading conditions. Creatine kinase-MB fractions exist in both skeletal and heart muscle but in different proportions. The mere presence of MB fraction isn't diagnostic but if markedly increased, as a fraction of the total CK, it makes myocardial injury more likely. CK-MB fractions do not stay elevated for more than 24 hours. Troponin I fractions are highly specific markers of myocardial cell death and could become the test of choice for myocardial infarction since they are unique to myocardial tissue and remain elevated for days after injury occurs. (**Ref. 23,** p. 14)

290. **(D)** Blood in the surgical field is suctioned off and is immediately mixed with an anticoagulant (heparin or citrate) and collected in a reservoir. It is then fed into a spinning plastic cone which, depending upon the rotational velocity, separates cellular and noncellular components. As this takes place, the supernatant is drawn off and a user-determined amount of saline is flushed

through and removed. The result is a concentrated product of mostly RBCs suspended in normal saline. Contamination can occur quite easily because solid matter in the surgical field, especially if adherent to RBCs, will not necessarily be washed off during processing. This is true for bacteria, some medications, and malignant cells. Activated clotting factors, free hemoglobin, and cellular debris are all fairly easily removed from such a system Microprocessor-controlled cell savers do have a processing cycle time of only 3 to 4 minutes before red cells are available for return to the patient. The risk of air embolism is reduced by the use of air detection alarms and shutoffs, but it is still a threat because air can be introduced depending upon how the cells are returned to the patient. (**Ref. 17,** pp. 93–123)

291. **(B)** Although all of the listed factors influence to some extent how much hemodilution occurs, the total red cell mass is the primary determinant of resulting hematocrit during CPB. Algorithms have been developed to try to predict blood volume from height, weight, and sex but are often inaccurate as a result of the effects of coexisting medical conditions, drug therapy, and other unclear factors. The formula below relates the effect of red cell volume on the resultant hematocrit on CPB.

$$\text{Predicted Hct on CPB}(\%) = \frac{BV \times Hct}{(BV + PPV + preCPB \text{ fluids})}$$
$$BV = \text{Blood volume} = \text{RBC mass} \times Hct$$
$$PPV = \text{Pump prime volume}$$

(**Ref. 17,** pp. 124–137)

292. **(A)** Aprotinin is a small protein molecule derived from beef lung tissue that recently received FDA approval for prophylactic use in patients at high risk for bleeding during cardiac surgery. Aprotinin has been shown in numerous studies to decrease postoperative chest tube drainage and to reduce the need for donor blood products. It is a protease inhibitor and as such has plasmin, kallikrein, and complement inhibiting activity. It also appears to protect platelets from the harmful effects of cardiopulmonary bypass. In contrast, neither steroids, opiates, antihistamines, nor prostaglandin inhibitors have anti-inflammatory effects of proven benefit during CPB. (**Ref. 23,** pp. 978–983)

293. (D) Surgical incision has been consistently shown to cause a decrease in the ACT. The mechanism by which this takes place is uncertain. Both hypothermia and hemodilution consistently prolong the ACT, and this is commonly observed after heparinization and the institution of cardiopulmonary bypass, which cause a further increase in the ACT despite no added heparin. Aprotinin, a serine protease inhibitor, with complex effects on coagulation, prolongs the celite ACT in the presence of heparin and has no consistent effect when heparin is absent. Protamine, in the absence of heparin, causes a prolongation of the ACT, suggesting that it has the potential to function as an anticoagulant in high doses. (**Ref. 17,** Chapter 14)

294. (C) Studies monitoring temperatures in multiple sites during simultaneous cooling and rewarming show that the sites to cool most rapidly are the same that warm the most rapidly. The order of sites rewarming from the fastest to slowest is: arterial cannula; myocardium; nasopharynx; brain; and rectum. The amount of blood flow to these sites is a major factor in the rate of change of temperature. Bladder temperatures depend upon urine output, and pulmonary artery temperatures are often reflective of the adjacent aortic cannula until pulmonary blood flow begins during partial bypass. (**Ref. 17,** pp. 592–595)

295. (C) To calculate the expected Hct of the patients on CPB, the volume of preoperative red blood cells must be estimated. Then, knowing the blood volume of the patient, the volume of the prime and preCPB IV fluids, minus urine output, the RBC volume is divided by the sum of these as shown below:

Hct on CPB = (RBC Volume)/(Blood Volume + IV Fluids + Pump Prime − Urine)

RBC Volume = Blood Volume × Hct

Blood Volume = Wt × 70 mL/kg (for adult females)

(**Ref. 17,** pp. 132–133)

296. **(E)** When a heart transplant is performed, all autonomic innervation is severed. Reflex responses to aortic or carotid baroreceptors or other indirectly mediated responses will not be observed. Instead, only the direct action of receptor activation on the myocardium will be seen. Norepinephrine will cause tachycardia and hypertension, atropine will not accelerate the sinus rate, and phenylephrine will increase blood pressure and not slow the heart rate. Pancuronium will have no effect on the heart rate. (**Ref. 42,** pp. 191–193)

297. **(D)** Invasive pressure measurement is subject to many influences from the site of monitoring in the patient all the way to the monitor itself. The type of signal processing algorithm used to determine where systolic, diastolic, and mean blood pressure are measured has greater influence, in general, on the systolic and diastolic pressure than on the mean pressure. Other noninvasive techniques differ even more in systolic and diastolic measurement but are quite close to a similar location when measured invasively. The dicrotic notch is detected only by invasive techniques and is not always present; the pulse pressure depends upon an accurate assessment of both systolic and diastolic components. It is fortunate that the mean blood pressure has probably the greatest relevance in organ blood flow. (**Ref. 37,** pp. 59–84)

298. **(D)** Cardioplegic solutions must be hypocalcemic because injury induced by free radicals is greatly enhanced by the presence of excess calcium. In fact, experimental evidence in animals suggests that the use of calcium channel blockers is beneficial to the ischemic heart. The retrograde distribution of cardioplegia differs from anterograde distribution in that the RV is not as well perfused. Anterograde is not as effective in the presence of severe proximal blockages without collateral flow, so that often a combination is sought in order to improve delivery to ischemic tissue. Collateral flow, when it exists, will cause a washout of cardioplegia and rewarming of the myocardium. This can be sufficient to endanger myocardial protection unless repeated doses of a cardioplegic solution are given. (**Ref. 17,** pp. 155–206)

299. **(E)** Histidine is the principal intracellular buffer responsible for maintaining a constant intracellular charge as temperature changes. This is characteristic of poikilotherms, and follows the

same changes that occur in the ratio of hydroxyl to hydrogen ions in water as temperature is changed. Alpha stat regulation refers to the maintenance of a constant total CO_2 as temperature falls; the alpha refers to the position of the imidazole group on histidine groups. In contrast to alpha stat, pH stat regulation is the addition of CO_2 during CPB to reduce the pH to normal (7.40) as temperature falls. As a result, total CO_2 increases and cerebral blood flow increases. This is characteristic of hibernation when animals hypoventilate and allow their body temperature to drop. There are no well-controlled studies showing important differences in outcome between both kinds of acid–base management, but the more convincing physiologic data tend to favor the use of alpha stat regulation. (**Ref. 17,** pp. 140–154)

300. **(A)** The success of chemical cardioplegia depends upon its composition and route of delivery. To be effective, it must buffer acidotic tissue and maintain alkalosis, reduce myocardial edema and minimize myocardial oxygen demands. Collateral blood flow and exposure to relatively warm environments (like room temperature) decrease the effectiveness of cold, chemical cardioplegia. Antecedent ischemia is common in patients with coronary artery disease, and further insult can lead to irreversible damage. Reperfusion injury occurs at the time of cross-clamp removal with the reintroduction of oxygen to the ischemic tissues. Injury is most likely mediated by free oxygen radicals, which attack normal contractile proteins and other cellular constituents, resulting in contractile dysfunction. The major source is probably the activated neutrophils, which generate free radicals as a component of the inflammatory response. Air embolism is uncommon and usually results in regional dysfunction and ST changes. It usually results in transient impairment only. The duration of cardiopulmonary bypass, within broad ranges, has little direct influence on the degree of myocardial injury. It does influence other program system responses, however, such as the degree of hemostasis. (**Ref. 17,** pp. 155–206)

301. **(C)** Terminal warm blood cardioplegia or "hot shot" cardioplegia has not been shown to affect the recovery of the conduction system or reduce the incidence of atrial fibrillation. Rewarming time is dependent upon the systemic temperature, flow rate on pump, and the size of the patient, and not on the use of "hot

shots." Both improved postischemic metabolic recovery and a sparing of the amount of high energy phosphates consumed after reperfusion occur with terminal warm blood cardioplegia. The fact that post-CPB function is improved reflects perhaps a reduction in reperfusion injury. (**Ref. 17,** pp. 155–206)

302. (A) Not enough is known about the effects of the cardiopulmonary bypass on pharmacokinetics to make sweeping generalizations, but some detailed studies have provided some insight. In general, the total drug concentration drops initially, due to hemodilution. Then the concentration slowly rises as redistribution occurs from the surrounding tissues. Drugs that are highly protein-bound are the most likely to undergo clinically important changes. Renal and hepatic clearance of drugs decreases. In vitro studies of binding to oxygenators suggests that large quantities of lipophilic drugs can be bound to membranes and to the polyurethane defoaming sponge in bubblers. It is doubtful whether these observations can be extrapolated directly to the clinical setting. (**Ref. 17,** pp. 207–220)

303. (B) Exposure to nonendothelialized surfaces, especially the huge surface areas occurring within oxygenators, are doubtless responsible for a characteristic inflammatory response that occurs despite the inhibition of thrombin because of the presence of large amounts of heparin. The lack of endothelium promotes platelet and leukocyte activation, contact activation via the Hageman factor, and activation of complement and plasmin. Recent evidence in humans during CPB suggests that the most significant stimulus might originate from the extrinsic pathway, that is, from the release of tissue thromboplastin from surgical incision and injury, disseminated during CPB. Although the type of oxygenator can influence the degree to which shear forces induce injury to red cells over time and the membranes are generally better tolerated for longer procedures than the bubblers, there is little evidence that the type of oxygenator makes a significant difference in the average case. Hypothermia does slow down the kinetics of enzyme-substrate interactions so that coagulation and platelet function would be expected to be transiently impaired. Hemodilution usually contributes to a drop in the levels of factors and platelets but not to levels that would independently cause abnormal hemostasis. (**Ref. 17,** pp. 233–248)

304. (C) In a survey of 284 incidents of air embolism during cardiopulmonary bypass, inattention to venous reservoir level and aortic root air during the administration of the cardioplegic solution were responsible for two-thirds of all events. Air embolism from an arterial line during flushing has been reported. There may be enough retrograde flow to reach the carotid artery under some circumstances, but this is a most unusual mechanism for clinically significant air embolism. An improper aortic cannulation site is a more likely cause of thrombotic or calcific embolism since the selection of an atherosclerotic segment for cannulation can dislodge intimal particulate matter. (**Ref. 17,** pp. 267–290)

305. (A) From the earliest days of extracorporeal technology, in the 1930s, to date, there have been continuously improving results from nonpulsatile perfusion. Studies that have attempted to compare outcomes and other measurable differences between pulsatile and nonpulsatile flow have shown inconsistent results, suggesting that there either are no significant differences or that studies differ in their definition and application of pulsatile flow in different patient populations. The technology to create a dynamic pulse pressure during CPB has existed for some time and could be marketed, but its added cost and complexity have made it unattractive to manufacturers. (**Ref. 17,** pp. 323–337)

306. (A) The two common sources are beef lung and pig intestines obtained from slaughterhouses. Heparin is a complex polyanionic polysaccharide that is actually a spectrum of molecules of widely varying molecular weight and potency. Heparin is an important constituent of tissue mast cells, and both these tissues are rich in this cell type. Accordingly, most authorities conclude that this is one of the principal sites of heparin synthesis and storage. Heparins in clinical use have not been produced by recombinant technology. Isolates of lower molecular weight have fewer in vitro side effects but have not been effective in vivo without significant postoperative bleeding complications. (**Ref. 17,** pp. 340–380)

307. (B) Because heparin is a principal component of tissue mast cells, it probably plays a role in nonimmunological defense, capillary angiogenesis, and lipid metabolism. Heparans, on the other hand, are a major related polysaccharide that is attached to the surface of vascular endothelium and binds to circulating AT III and potentiates thrombin inhibition. Heparans are most likely the natural AT III agonist in humans. Unfractionated molecular weights of heparin average 15,000 Daltons and commonly range from 3,000 to over 40,000 Daltons. The variability depends upon the animal and tissue source. The degree of conformational change induced in AT III varies from lot to lot as well, resulting in variations in potency per weight. It is therefore important to speak of heparin in terms of units of activity rather than milligrams. Heparin has the lowest pKa of any large molecule in the body, making it a highly acidic molecule. (**Ref. 17,** pp. 340–380)

308. **(A)** In the majority of patients a 300 U/kg dose of heparin, concentration in whole blood of 3 U/mL, measured by protamine titration, and/or an ACT > 300 sec is sufficient for safe initiation of cardiopulmonary bypass. Exceptions do occur in the following ways. Some patients can be described as "heparin-resistant" because with a standard dose of heparin their ACT does not rise above 300 sec. Such a patient may be AT III deficient and could be treated with additional heparin or by the administration of AT III (such as FFP or AT III concentrates, which are very expensive). The whole blood concentration of heparin does not indicate that the drug's effect is adequate. A "resistant" patient may actually need a much higher concentration of heparin. No one has established what the safe lower limits are for ACTs, nor are there likely to be any studies in humans defining where this threshold exists. The value of 480 sec commonly quoted includes a rather arbitrary "safety" margin factored in by researchers, allowing for the variability in response among patients. Prolonged CPB usually requires redosing heparin to maintain a certain level or prolongation of the ACT, suggesting that even under hypothermic conditions the anticoagulant effect of heparin can diminish. Both the aPTT and PT become indefinitely prolonged with the large doses of heparin used, rendering these tests useless for heparin monitoring during CPB. (**Ref. 17,** pp. 340–380)

309. **(E)** Prior heparin therapy binds AT III and can depress levels for days following discontinuation of treatment. Severe thrombocytosis and eosinophilia increase resistance by uncertain mechanisms. The association of heparin resistance with nitroglycerin therapy has been observed by some but not by all authors. Sepsis may cause an acquired AT III deficiency, which has been observed in endocarditis and hypercoagulable states such as DIC. (**Ref. 17,** pp. 340–380)

310. **(B)** Protamine has two distinct binding sites. One is arginine-rich and therefore strongly cationic and binds heparin, the other is responsible for the anticoagulant effect of protamine. The relationship between heparin and the amount of protamine required for neutralization is variable and in vitro testing differs from in vivo testing in this regard. It is wise, therefore, not to rely only on fixed ratios but on titration, based on clinical factors and supported by in vitro testing. NPH stands for neutral protamine Hagedorn insulin, protamine is added to retard the absorption of insulin. (**Ref. 17,** pp. 381–406)

311. **(C)** Because this patient needs this procedure because of the risk of progression to permanent myocardial injury, there are better options than stopping at this point. Some have argued that an ACT of 300 is probably safe for the majority of patients, but this patient, most likely as a result of previous heparin therapy, is now resistant to heparin. Giving additional heparin is usually effective, suggesting the presence of competitive inhibitors or a change in AT III activity. Antithrombin III tests (AT III activity and antigen) are not useful under these circumstances because both are usually diminished. Unless extremely low, it is usually not possible to distinguish an acquired from a congenital deficiency. A low level also does not exclude other reasons such as inhibitors. AT III tests are thus not useful. Plasma contains AT III and giving FFP usually provides enough AT III activity to allow the ACT to rise significantly. Recombinant AT III does not exist; pooled AT III concentrates that have been specially treated to reduce viral transmission are available from several drug companies but are extremely expensive. There are no studies evaluating the risk/benefit of AT III concentrates under these conditions, and obtaining the drug quickly would be difficult. (**Ref. 23,** pp. 964–966)

312. **(E)** The range of reported reactions to protamine is quite varied and few studies on the mechanisms exist, in part because a predictable animal model has not yet been found. Rapid administration of protamine frequently is associated with hypotension. The role of histamine in this hypotension is suggested by studies in

humans and dogs, and seems related to the rate of administration. Some authors have attempted to show a direct myocardial depressant effect of protamine, but this isn't clear. Anaphylaxis is a rare complication that has been documented only in diabetics on NPH or protamine–zinc insulin preparations. Presumably IgE was formed from prior exposure to protamine, but this is difficult to prove and among patients with prior exposure the frequency of reactions appears quite uncommon. Catastrophic pulmonary edema with sudden, acute right heart failure and sometimes pulmonary edema alone is another consistently reported phenomenon associated with protamine. It has been suggested that this is an anaphylactoid reaction caused by IgG and complement activation. Delayed reactions have also been reported (10 to 30 min after administration). (**Ref. 17,** pp. 381–406)

313. **(E)** An IABP can cause limb ischemia by obstruction to flow, both at the site of entry into the vascular system and at the location of the balloon (for example, obstruction of the celiac vessels leading to mesenteric ischemia). Embolization of cholesterol from the aortic intima and of gas from a ruptured or leaking helium balloon can occur. Many hemodynamic monitors are not capable of correctly identifying systolic and diastolic blood pressure from a patient with a balloon pump in place, due to the unusual arterial wave forms resulting from balloon inflation during aortic valve closure. Dissection is caused by direct injury during the placement of the balloon. (**Ref. 17,** pp. 699–701)

314. **(A)** Prolonged aortic cross-clamping defines the period during which the myocardium is ischemic. When this time exceeds 2 hours, the likelihood of stunning or more significantly, less reversible injuries begin to increase even under optimal conditions of protection. Any time the ventricular muscle is cut to remove lesions, a clot, or an aneurysm, the function of that muscle will be adversely affected. Mitral valve replacement has a greater negative impact on ventricular function than repair because the contribution of the papillary muscles to ejection is significant. During replacement, the chordae are severed and ventricular geometry changes. In addition, patients with mitral regurgitation suffer afterload mismatch with valve replacement, and this contributes to poor function. (**Ref. 17,** pp. 766–767)

315. (A) This patient has most likely suffered an acute, severe reaction to protamine, characterized by sudden increase in pulmonary vascular resistance, acute right heart failure, and hypotension. An acutely afterloaded right ventricle dilates and becomes very dependent upon systolic coronary blood flow for survival. It is the mean aortic pressure–mean RVEDP gradient that determines the driving pressure for perfusion. Therefore, stopping the protamine and administering a potent catecholamine to increase mean aortic pressure is likely to be of benefit. In addition, an immediate return to CPB may also be indicated if initial attempts at recovery of right heart function fail. Thus a bolus of heparin, sufficient for the safe reinstitution of CPB is also wise. Although effective in reducing PVR, prostaglandins are not specific to the lung, and systemic vasodilation occurs as well, so that a vasoconstrictor is still necessary. CaCl is unlikely to be potent enough to reverse the hemodynamic predicament of the right heart. Interestingly enough, there are a number of case reports on the acute reversal of this reaction to protamine by the administration of heparin. It has been suggested that the mechanism is related to circulating free heparin–protamine complexes. (**Ref. 23,** pp. 973–977)

316. (C) Most antiarrhythmic drugs are also negative inotropes to varying degrees, but this is not the mechanism of arrhythmia suppression. Most drugs act by decreasing automaticity of the myocardial tissue by increasing the threshold required for depolarization. Antiarrhythmics almost uniformly decrease conduction velocity in atrial and/or ventricular tissue. Such drugs can also become proarrhythmic under conditions of decremental conduction and unidirectional block. (**Ref. 22,** pp. 929–930; **Ref. 7,** pp. 779–782)

317. (A) There are numerous case reports of pulmonary hypertensive crises following mitral valve surgery, transplantation, and pulmonary embolectomy. The treatment depends upon the severity of impairment of RV function, but the goals are all the same: Maintain RV perfusion pressure, lower SVR, decrease RV preload, and increase stroke volume in both RV and LV. Vasectomized patients are not clearly at increased risk for hypertensive reactions based on available data, nor are diabetics. Therefore routine prophylactic strategies are not indicated. (**Ref. 23,** pp. 973–977)

318. **(C)** Adenosine is an important endogenous nucleoside that acts locally to depress SA and AV node activity, to regulate myocardial metabolism via coronary vasodilation, and to blunt catechol-mediated stimulation. It is effective in most forms of VT, can make hypotension worse by slowing heart rate and enhancing vasodilation, and can make ischemia worse. Adenosine is indicated in the termination of AV nodal re-entrant SVT, and it is used routinely with thallium perfusion scanning to measure coronary flow reserve. (**Ref. 23,** p. 701)

319. **(A)** A CVP is very useful for the detection of AV dyssynchrony, such as occurs in heart block, junctional rhythm, and atrial flutter or fibrillation. Not only does atrial mean pressure change but very distinctive and often diagnostic changes are seen in the waveforms, allowing rapid detection and diagnosis even during electrocautery. For the same reason atrial capture and proper timing of pacing can be monitored using the CVP waveform. The CVP is an excellent estimate of RVEDP, the filling pressure of the RV, so long as no tricuspid stenosis exists. Severe MR and elevated LVEDP can eventually be reflected in elevations in the CVP, but there are so many exceptions and conditional requirements for this to occur reliably that the CVP should never be assumed to provide information regarding most events on the left side of the heart. (**Ref. 27,** pp. 147–196)

320. **(E)** Atherosclerosis commonly causes plaque formation in the arterial tree. Proximal stenoses are common and should be looked for by comparing, for example, cuff pressures bilaterally before deciding which radial artery to monitor. Systemic vasodilation alters the conduction of vibrations from the central aorta to the periphery in such a way that some components of invasive pressure waveforms are altered more than others. For similar reasons, altering the filtering frequency of the monitor from one site to another or having different resonant frequencies influences the measurement of pressures. Techniques such as oscillometry or auscultatory pressure measurements often result in differences attributable to different end points (i.e., a Korotkoff sound is not necessarily equivalent to oscillometric or invasive markers of the pulse contour). (**Ref. 8,** pp. 93–115)

321. (A) TEE probes are large and interfere with airway management, induction, emergence, and extubation. Therefore, at these times TEE cannot provide useful information. Artifact interference occurs as a result of electrocautery to the position of the heart relative to the esophagus, to the intracardiac septum, and in the presence of bundle branch block. Lack of specificity exists in the detection of ischemia because of the tethering effect of the heart (normal tissue surrounding ischemic tissue appears to move abnormally), scar, changes in afterload, and the presence of stunned myocardium. TEE is very sensitive in detecting air particles. (**Ref. 23,** pp. 370–371)

13

Anesthesia for Vascular Surgery

DIRECTIONS (Questions 322–340): For each of the questions or incomplete answers below, **one** or **more** of the answers or completions are correct. Select

- **A.** if only 1, 2, and 3 are correct
- **B.** if only 1 and 3 are correct
- **C.** if only 2 and 4 are correct
- **D.** if only 4 is correct
- **E.** if all are correct

---

322. Cerebral ischemia can occur as a result of
1. hypotension
2. embolization of the distal intracranial vasculature
3. a "steal" phenomenon (i.e., a diversion of blood from intracranial pathways to extracranial sites)
4. maximal dilation of normal intracranial vessels at the expense of those areas supplied by diseased vessels

323. The indications for surgical intervention for carotid artery disease include
1. the presence of a carotid bruit
2. verified stenosis of greater than 75% to 80% with or without symptoms
3. recent acute stroke, less than 6 weeks before planned surgical intervention
4. presence of cerebral ischemic symptoms with high-grade carotid stenosis

324. The symptoms of cerebral ischemia secondary to carotid disease can be classified as
1. reversible ischemic neurologic deficits
2. acute stroke
3. transient ischemic attacks
4. subclavian steal syndrome

325. The major anesthetic goals for carotid endarterectomy include
1. protecting the brain and heart from ischemia
2. ensuring adequate cerebral and myocardial blood flow
3. evaluating the neurologic status when carotid endarterectomy is done under regional anesthesia
4. ensuring adequate myocardial perfusion by raising central venous pressure above intracranial pressure while maintaining a constant mean arterial pressure

326. Cerebral perfusion can be directly influenced by which of the following variables?
1. CVP
2. ICP
3. MAP
4. hemoglobin level

327. Which of the following statements is (are) accurate regarding the potential advantages of regional anesthesia for carotid endarterectomy?
1. superior ability to assess neurologic status
2. higher incidence of perioperative myocardial infarction because the awake patient is more anxious
3. increased cost savings resulting from shorter ICU stays
4. decreased blood pressure variations perioperatively

188 / 13: Anesthesia for Vascular Surgery

328. Which of the following describe(s) a deep cervical plexus block?
   1. it involves the dermatome levels C_3, C_4, and C_5
   2. its landmarks include Chassaignac's tubercle, the sternocleidomastoid muscle, and the mastoid process
   3. the spinous processes of the appropriate cervical vertebrae are targeted
   4. possible complications include total spinal, intravascular injection, and Horner's syndrome

329. Which of the following volatile anesthetics has the most favorable cerebral metabolic effects with respect to protecting the brain from ischemia?
   1. halothane
   2. enflurane
   3. cyclopropane
   4. isoflurane

330. Patients who have had bilateral carotid endarterectomies may be especially vulnerable to respiratory depressants postoperatively because
   1. their airway is more likely to become compromised by hematoma formation if there is contralateral scarring
   2. general anesthesia is required for the second carotid endarterectomy
   3. they are more likely to have recurrent laryngeal nerve damage
   4. there is potential for bilateral carotid body dysfunction and these patients could lose compensatory mechanisms in response to hypoxia

331. The different types of aortic aneurysms include
   1. fusiform
   2. atherosclerotic
   3. saccular
   4. syphilitic

332. The DeBakey Type II aortic dissection involves
   1. an intimal tear in the ascending aorta and the dissection usually extends throughout the aorta
   2. an intimal tear in the proximal descending aorta and the dissection extends to the abdominal aorta

3. an intimal tear in the descending aorta without dissection
4. an intimal tear occurs in the ascending aorta and the dissection is limited to the ascending aorta

333. Upon cross-clamping the thoracic aorta, the hemodynamic change(s) that occur include(s)
    1. increased afterload
    2. hypotension distally
    3. hypertension proximally
    4. dramatic decreases in heart rate and cardiac output in laboratory animals with normal hearts

334. The ischemic damage to the spinal cord, after cross-clamping the descending aorta
    1. is similar to that of anterior spinal syndrome
    2. typically involves loss of motor function and pinprick sensation
    3. vibratory and position sense are usually preserved
    4. may involve the occlusion of the artery of Adamkiewicz

335. Sodium nitroprusside used during aortic surgery
    1. rapidly controls proximal hypertension
    2. increases the amount of right-to-left pulmonary shunting
    3. inhibits pulmonary hypoxic vasoconstriction
    4. increases the cerebral spinal fluid pressure

336. Measures to help prevent postaortic-clamp paraplegia include
    1. left heart bypass
    2. cerebral spinal fluid drainage
    3. right atrial to femoral artery bypass
    4. routine use of nitroprusside to vasodilate and thus increase blood flow to the spinal cord

337. Adequate preoperative cardiac evaluation for patients with severe peripheral vascular occlusive disease is essential. A method of accurately evaluating left ventricular function and myocardium at risk for ischemia in patients with disabling lower extremity claudication could be
    1. 12-lead ECG
    2. dobutamine echocardiogram
    3. stress testing according to standard Bruce protocols
    4. dipyridamole thallium scan

338. A patient is undergoing an abdominal aortic aneurysm resection. Following an estimated blood loss of 12,000 mL, the patient develops a hemorrhagic diathesis. Possible causes and possible treatments include
   1. residual heparinization—administer protamine
   2. dilutional thrombocytopenia—transfuse platelets
   3. hemolytic transfusion reaction—stop transfusion, maintain urine flow with fluids and diuretics, investigate
   4. DIC—administer Amicar (epsilon-aminocaproic acid)

339. During anesthesia for carotid endarterectomy
   1. patients should be hyperventilated to a CO_2 of approximately 25 torr
   2. stump pressure measurements correlate well with cerebral blood flow measurements and with EEG findings at the time of cross-clamping
   3. thiobarbiturates should be administered prior to cross-clamping, because they will suppress EEG activity during the entire period of occlusion
   4. deep and superficial cervical plexus block provides an attractive alternative to general anesthesia

340. Abdominal aortic aneurysm surgery
   1. may be associated with acute renal failure if urine flow is not maintained
   2. is an indication for invasive arterial blood pressure and pulmonary artery pressure monitoring
   3. is often associated with a rise of 7 or more mm Hg of pulmonary capillary wedge pressure with application of the aortic cross-clamp. This may indicate left ventricular dysfunction or incipient ischemia
   4. should not be done under epidural anesthesia because of the risk of peridural hematoma from intraoperative heparinization

DIRECTIONS (Questions 341–344): Each of the questions or incomplete statements below is followed by five suggested answers or completions. Select the **one** that is best in each case.

341. Probably the most reliable method for monitoring cerebral blood flow during carotid endarterectomy is
    A. carotid artery stump pressures
    B. processed electroencephalogram
    C. unprocessed electroencephalogram
    D. jugular venous oxygen saturation
    E. somatosensory evoked potentials

342. Cerebral protection provided by barbiturates during carotid artery endarterectomy is characterized by all of the following EXCEPT
    A. protective in global ischemia
    B. initially produces slowing of, or an isoelectric EEG
    C. may induce cardiovascular instability in high doses
    D. the protective effects are temporary
    E. protective in focal ischemia

343. The optimal site for the placement of a single arterial catheter for proximal blood pressure monitoring during descending thoracoabdominal aneurysm repair is the
    A. right femoral artery
    B. left radial artery
    C. left axillary artery
    D. right radial artery
    E. left femoral artery

344. You are called to the recovery room to evaluate a patient who has had a carotid artery endarterectomy. The patient is in moderate, but worsening respiratory distress. Examination reveals a swollen and tense neck wound. The pulse oximeter shows 90% saturation. After providing supplemental oxygen, your next course of action is
- **A.** induce anesthesia with barbiturates, give succinylcholine, and intubate the patient
- **B.** send an arterial blood sample to the laboratory because you suspect the pulse oximeter of malfunction
- **C.** order a chest x-ray to rule out a pneumothorax
- **D.** perform an indirect laryngoscopy to examine the vocal cords for signs of recurrent laryngeal nerve damage
- **E.** open the wound immediately and return the patient to the operating room for surgical exploration

Anesthesia for Vascular Surgery

Answers and Discussion

The authors have made every effort to thoroughly verify the answers to the questions that appear on the preceding pages. As in any text, however, some inaccuracies and ambiguities may occur. If in doubt, please consult the indicated reference. When no page number(s) are cited, the reference is to a journal article or to a refresher course lecture that should be read in its entirety.

The Editors

322. (E) Atherosclerosis of the major extracranial arteries can produce cerebral ischemia by any one of three mechanisms, or by a combination thereof: (1) marked reduction in blood flow, either by stenosis or occlusion of a vessel responsible for supplying blood to the brain or reduction in blood flow by systemic hypotension; (2) distal embolization by atheromatous debris released from an ulcerated plaque; and (3) diversion of blood flow from intracranial pathways to extracranial sites creating what is known as a *steal phenomenon* (e.g., subclavian steal syndrome). Another example of the steal phenomenon is known as *intracerebral steal,* when blood flow to ischemic areas is diverted from these ischemic regions to nonischemic areas of the brain where the blood vessels are able to dilate under the influence of potent vasodilators (e.g., hypercarbia). This diversion occurs because the stenosed vessels are already maximally dilated and therefore unable to respond further to the effects of the vasodilators. (**Ref. 32,** pp. 1704–1705, 1713)

323. (C) Performing a carotid endarterectomy in an asymptomatic patient is somewhat controversial. Chambers and Norris reported that if the degree of stenosis was found to be less than 75%, the annual risk of stroke was less than 1%. If the stenosis was found to be greater than 75%, the annual risk of stroke increased to 5%. The perioperative stroke rate for carotid endarterectomy has been reported to be about 3.7% in asymptomatic patients. Many centers are therefore not recommending endarterectomy in asymptomatic patients unless the underlying stenosis is greater than 75% to 80%. The mere presence of a carotid bruit is not an indication for surgical intervention unless the underlying stenosis is greater than 75% to 80%, an ulcerated plaque is present, or there are symptoms indicative of carotid disease.

Transient ischemic attacks typically reflect an underlying stenosis of 70% or more or the presence of an ulcerated plaque. The stroke risk in patients who have had TIAs is approximately 4% to 6% per year. The annual risk of recurrent stroke without endarterectomy is about 5% to 10%, carrying with it a mortality of 20% to 30%. Indications for carotid endarterectomy in symptomatic patients is therefore more clear.

Patients who have experienced a stroke within 6 weeks before surgery have a 20-fold increase in the risk of intraoperative cerebral ischemia. In general, it is recommended that carotid endarterectomy not be performed for at least 4 to 6 weeks after an acute stroke. (**Ref. 25,** pp. 334–336)

324. (A) Symptoms of cerebral ischemia are consistent with central nervous system abnormalities. These abnormalities can typically be classified into any one of three categories: (1) transient ischemic attacks (TIAs), which are CNS events that last less than 24 hours and totally resolve; (2) strokes, which are events that last longer than 24 hours and may not totally resolve; and (3) reversible ischemic neurologic deficits (RINDS), which are CNS events that last more than 24 hours but less than 3 weeks and totally resolve. Symptoms consistent with upper extremity ischemia are not typically a result of cerebral ischemia. In fact, the more common situation—as in the case of the *subclavian steal syndrome*—is when the increased demands of an exercised upper extremity causes a diversion of blood flow away from the cerebral vasculature to the involved upper extremity. This redistribution of blood flow is at the expense of the cerebral vasculature, thus creating or worsening areas of the brain at risk of ischemia. (**Ref. 32, p. 1705; Ref. 25,** pp. 334–335)

325. (A) The major goals of anesthetic management for carotid endarterectomy are to provide a pain-free patient, to facilitate the surgical procedure, and to minimize the perioperative morbidity and mortality. With respect to minimizing perioperative morbidity and mortality, it must be appreciated that the great majority of perioperative morbidity and mortality results from myocardial and/or cerebral ischemia. In attempting to decrease myocardial oxygen requirements, there is a need to decrease heart rate, blood pressure, and myocardial contractility. To maintain or increase cerebral perfusion pressure requires an increase in mean arterial pressure above the normal brain autoregulatory threshold. In accomplishing this, it is essential to avoid hypotension by a reduction in cardiac output and/or systemic vascular resistance. When regional anesthesia is chosen for carotid endarterectomy in the awake patient, the patient must be able to respond to commands to allow an adequate assessment of the neurologic status during the operation. Oversedation, panic, or confusion can render this assessment useless. A fine line must be drawn between adequate anxiolysis and oversedation. (**Ref. 37,** p. 106)

326. (A) One of the primary anesthetic considerations during carotid endarterectomy is the maintenance of a critical perfusion pressure. Cerebral blood flow is normally autoregulated between mean arterial pressures of 40 to 160 mm Hg, giving a cerebral blood flow of 40 to 60 mL/100 g/min. Cerebral perfusion pressure is defined as the mean arterial pressure (MAP) minus intracranial pressure (ICP) or central venous pressure (CVP), depending on which is higher. From this it can be reasoned that as ICP increases, there must be a compensatory increase in the MAP to maintain CPP. It is important also that the autoregulatory curve

for CBF may undergo a right or left shift depending on whether the patient is chronically hyper- or hypotensive. (**Ref. 25,** pp. 339–340)

327. (B) Although there is some controversy surrounding these issues, proponents of regional anesthesia claim, and are supported by various studies, that there is a better ability to assess the patient's neurologic status, a lower overall incidence of perioperative myocardial infarction, a reduced incidence of blood pressure variance, and a reduced stay in the intensive care unit (thus reducing the hospital costs). Investigators have found it advantageous to conduct a trial of temporary carotid artery occlusion to determine whether there is any change in the neurologic status during the clamping period. If there are no symptoms, there is no need for shunt placement. Carotid endarterectomy under regional anesthesia grants the opportunity to assess the early onset of anginal symptoms. With respect to perioperative blood pressure lability, there are studies that both support and refute the contention that there is less hemodynamic instability when regional anesthesia is chosen for carotid surgery. In one study looking at the cost benefits of regional anesthesia for this procedure, it was found that the patients who received general anesthesia stayed two days longer in the hospital overall and for approximately one additional day in the intensive care unit. (**Ref. 25,** pp. 342–347)

328. (C) Deep cervical plexus blockade involves placement of block needles at the transverse processes of C_2, C_3, and C_4. Landmarks include the mastoid process, the sternocleidomastoid muscle, and Chassaignac's tubercle. The C_2 transverse process is usually one finger-breadth below the mastoid process along the line created between the mastoid process and Chassaignac's tubercle. The transverse processes of C_3 and C_4 can be located by progressing down that line at 2-cm intervals. At each location, 4 to 7 mL of the local anesthetic of choice is deposited after careful aspiration. An alternative single injection technique may also be used. A line is drawn laterally from the superior border of the thyroid cartilage to the point at which it intersects the groove between the anterior and middle scalene muscles posterior to the posterior border of the sternocleidomastoid muscle. The needle is then advanced perpendicular to all planes until paresthesias are elicited or the transverse process is contacted. Fifteen to 30 mL of local anesthetic is deposited. Possible complications of the deep cervical plexus blockade include intravascular injection, total spinal, and Horner's syndrome. (**Ref. 25,** pp. 345–347)

329. (D) Cerebral blood flow (CBF) is normally 40 to 50 mL/100 g/min. The EEG amplitude begins to diminish in the unprotected or anesthetized brain when the CBF decreases to 16 to 20 mL/100 g/min. At a CBF of 12 to 16 mL/100 g/min there is flattening of the EEG, and at a CBF of less than 10 mL/100 g/min cellular death begins. Critical cerebral blood flow (CCBF) is defined as the blood flow below which cerebral ischemia is evident on the EEG. For patients receiving halothane and nitrous oxide at normocarbia, the CCBF is approximately 20 mL/100 g/min. With enflurane and nitrous oxide, the CCBF is 15 mL/100 g/min. Finally, patients under isoflurane and nitrous oxide anesthesia tolerate a CCBF of 10 mL/100 g/min. Isoflurane is the only one of the foregoing inhalation anesthetics that produces an isoelectric EEG at 2 MAC, and it appears to have a cerebral metabolic profile not unlike that of barbiturates. (**Ref. 25,** pp. 347–348)

330. (D) The carotid bodies function to stimulate the respiratory center in the medulla. Stimulation is incited by a rise in $PaCO_2$ or in H^+ concentration. The carotid bodies are also stimulated when there is a decrease in the PaO_2. Patients who have undergone bilateral carotid endarterectomies suffer loss of carotid body responsiveness to hypoxia and therefore are more vulnerable to respiratory depressants. The compensatory mechanisms that respond to hypoxia are no longer intact, making medications such as narcotics and other sedatives more likely to produce profound hypoxia. (**Ref. 25,** p. 355)

331. (E) Aortic aneurysms can be classified on the basis of either morphology, location, or etiology. Morphologically, aneurysms can be differentiated into fusiform, saccular, and dissecting aneurysms. Classification by etiology includes atherosclerotic, syphilitic, and mycotic aneurysms. Typically, the aneurysms that are the result of atherosclerosis are fusiform, and the syphilitic ones are saccular. Classification on the basis of location include ascending (between the annulus of the aortic valve and the innominate artery), transverse (arising from the arch), descending (distal to the left subclavian artery), and thoracoabdominal aortic aneurysms (beginning in the descending aorta but extending distally beyond the diaphragm). (**Ref. 25,** pp. 364–369)

332. (D) According to the DeBakey Classification of Aortic Dissections, the Type I dissecting aortic aneurysm begins with the intimal tear in the ascending aorta and extends throughout the aorta. The Type II dissecting aneurysm begins with an intimal tear in the ascending aorta but extends no further than the ascending aorta. Type III aortic dissections begin with the intimal tear in the descending thoracic aorta, just distal to the origin of the left subclavian artery, and progresses distally. (**Ref. 25,** pp. 368–370)

333. (A) Placing a cross-clamp on the descending thoracic aorta typically increases the mean arterial pressure proximal to the clamp by approximately 40%. The mean arterial pressure distal to the clamp decreases to approximately 15% of the preclamp values, with a range between 11 and 26 mm Hg. Central venous pressure increases about 2 mm Hg. In laboratory models coronary blood flow has been shown to increase approximately 40%. Interestingly enough, there are minimal changes in heart rate or cardiac output in laboratory animals with normal hearts. A slow release of the aortic clamp is essential to allow time for compensatory measures to be taken to minimize declamp hypotension. This is thought to be due to a low systemic vascular resistance as well as to the release of vasodilating metabolites that have accumulated during the clamp interval. (**Ref. 25,** pp. 377–379)

334. (E) In a review of 360 patients undergoing descending thoracic aorta repair, Livesay et al. reported an operative mortality of 11.7% and an incidence of paraplegia of 6.5%. The clinical presentation of patients who have suffered ischemic damage to the spinal cord after such a repair is similar to that seen in the anterior spinal syndrome. The latter occurs after occlusion of the radicularis magna anterior artery, also known as the artery of Adamkiewicz. This syndrome involves a loss of motor function and pinprick sensation, whereas vibratory and position sense are usually intact. The artery of Adamkiewicz has a variable origin ranging from T_5 to L_5. The variability of this artery's origin makes predicting postoperative spinal cord ischemic sequelae difficult. (**Ref. 25,** pp. 379–383)

335. (E) Sodium nitroprusside is commonly used to control the proximal hypertension that is created when cross-clamping the aorta. The rate of infusion should not exceed 6 µg/kg/min to avoid the possibility of cyanide toxicity. Many systemic vasodilators have been shown to inhibit hypoxic pulmonary vasoconstriction (HPV) and therefore increase the degree of right-to-left intrapulmonary shunting. Examples of drugs that have been shown to inhibit HPV include nitroglycerin, nitroprusside, dobutamine, several calcium antagonists, and many B_2 agonists. (**Ref. 25,** pp. 385–386)

336. (A) The blood flow to the spinal cord decreases dramatically (84% to 90%) when the descending thoracic aorta is clamped. The methods employed to ameliorate this situation and partially restore blood flow to the cord include the placement of vascular shunts, left heart bypass, mild hypothermia, steroids, and cerebrospinal fluid drainage. Sodium nitroprusside has been reported to have the effect of increasing the cerebrospinal fluid pressure and of decreasing spinal cord blood flow during aortic cross-clamping, resulting in an increased rate of paraplegia in dogs. (**Ref. 25,** pp. 385–386)

337. (C) Preoperative cardiac evaluation of the patients undergoing vascular surgery is essential. A typical study for evaluating the patients for underlying ischemic heart disease and decreased cardiac function is an exercise stress test. In this particular subset of patients with severe peripheral vascular occlusive disease, many patients are not able to satisfactorily complete the standard exercise tests due to severe claudication. Under these circumstances, the use of the stress test is inadequate. Dipyridamole thallium and dobutamine echocardiography have been used in these patients to evaluate both left ventricular function and to identify a myocardium potentially at risk for ischemia. (**Ref. 25,** pp. 369–373)

338. (A) The intraoperative fluid and blood loss begins with the skin incision. With the degree of bowel manipulation involved in aortic surgery, there is a considerable degree of "third spacing." Blood loss during aortic surgery is frequently the result of venous bleeding due to the close proximity of the venous system to the arteries typically involved in aortoiliac surgery. After the release of the aortic cross-clamp following aneurysmectomy, it is not unusual for the patient to require volume resuscitation with crystalloids and/or blood products. If, five to ten minutes after removal of the clamp, hypotension persists in the absence of obvious surgical bleeding, sources of occult bleeding must be considered. As blood loss continues, coagulopathies eventually develop with dilutional thrombocytopenia usually occurring first. This can become important at platelet counts of less than 50,000 to 100,000 platelets/mm^3. The treatment consists of the administration of platelets.

Other causes of continued bleeding in the patient undergoing aneurysmectomy include residual heparinization and the occurrence of a possible transfusion reaction. Clinically, if after the repair has been completed and there are no signs of ongoing bleeding, reversal of heparin is not required. If there is continued "oozing," the reversal or additional reversal of heparin with protamine may be required after determining the ACT. Under general anesthesia, the only signs of a transfusion reaction may be hemoglobinuria, bleeding diatheses, or hypotension. Treatment includes the discontinuation of the transfusion, the maintenance and alkalinization of urine, and various laboratory studies assessing the effects on the hematologic and coagulation systems.

Epsilon aminocaproic acid (EACA) inhibits the formation of plasmin and attenuates fibrinolysis. EACA should not be used as a treatment for disseminated intravascular coagulation because it blocks the fibrinolytic system, whereas in DIC the coagulation system is activated. There is a risk of diffuse thrombosis in this situation. (**Ref. 25,** pp. 559–561; **Ref. 32,** p. 1480)

339. **(D)** Deep and superficial cervical plexus block provides an attractive alternative to general anesthesia. Proponents of regional anesthesia claim and are supported by various studies that there is a better ability to assess the patient's neurologic status, a lower overall incidence of perioperative myocardial infarction, a reduced incidence of blood pressure variations, and a reduced stay in the intensive care unit, thus reducing the hospital costs.

Normocarbia is advocated. Hypoventilation has been suggested in the past. Subsequent investigations, however, indicate that hypercarbia could produce a "steal phenomenon." Hypercarbia, in this situation, would induce vasodilation of normal vessels, thus diverting the much needed blood flow away from the ischemic areas—which are unable to dilate further—to well-perfused areas. Hyperventilation has been implicated in exacerbating cerebral ischemia by causing vasoconstriction in the preexisting ischemic areas and further decreasing cerebral blood flow to those areas. Stump pressures, though widely used, do not reliably correlate with CBF measurements nor do they correlate well with EEG changes. Neither the stump pressure nor the EEG may accurately assess the adequacy of cerebral perfusion in patients who have suffered a stroke or have a reversible ischemic neurologic deficit (RIND). (**Ref. 25,** pp. 343–348; **Ref. 32,** pp. 1712–1713)

340. **(A)** Descending thoracic aneurysms and infrarenal and suprarenal abdominal aortic aneurysms will require aortic cross-clamping either above or near the renal arteries, therefore predisposing the patient to renal ischemic damage. Other factors that are associated with acute renal failure after aortic surgery include massive transfusion, preoperative hypotension, and plaque embolization to the renal arteries. Protective measures include maintenance of intravascular volume and cardiac output, avoidance of hypotension, and the use of diuretics when indicated. To accurately assess all these parameters as well as to optimize hemodynamics, aortic reconstructive surgery frequently requires the use of invasive monitors in the form of an arterial line and a pulmonary artery catheter.

    Though somewhat controversial, epidural anesthesia is not contraindicated. Cases of peridural hematoma from any central conduction block are exceedingly rare, unless the patient has a severe, preexisting coagulopathy. Heparinization more than one hour after the placement of the epidural catheter is not dangerous. (**Ref. 25,** pp. 386–387; **Ref. 32,** pp. 1718–1719)

341. **(E)** The methods used to monitor the adequacy of cerebral circulation include stump pressures, jugular venous oxygen saturation, xenon washout, processed EEG, unprocessed EEG, near-infrared monitoring, conjunctival oxygen tension, Doppler ultrasound, ophthalmoplethysmography, and evoked potentials. All these methods have various drawbacks and have, to some degree, been associated with both false negatives and false positives. A possible exception to this might be somatosensory-evoked potentials. Auditory- and visual-evoked potentials are of little value in this area. Stump pressures as a measure of collateral cerebral flow correlates poorly with EEG findings and neither EEG nor stump

pressures assess the adequacy of cerebral perfusion in stroke patients or RIND patients. Neither jugular venous oxygen saturation nor xenon washout is indicative of focal cerebral ischemia and reflect only global perfusion. Conjunctival oxygen saturation, supraorbital plethysmography, and ophthalmoplethysmography assess only ophthalmic artery flow and therefore infarcts in other areas can go undetected. (**Ref. 25,** pp. 348–350)

342. **(A)** Barbiturates have been reported to be somewhat protective in focal cerebral ischemia, but there has been little or no evidence that they provide any protection against global ischemia. Barbiturates given just prior to clamping the carotid produce a slowing of the EEG or an isoelectric EEG, although the EEG usually returns to baseline within 10 minutes to an hour. High doses of barbiturate have been given to patients who were undergoing normothermic cardiopulmonary bypass, and they seemed to provide some protection. These doses, however, are too large to be considered in patients undergoing carotid endarterectomy because hemodynamic instability can result from the cardiovascular effects of such large doses. (**Ref. 25,** pp. 350–351)

343. **(D)** Monitoring for aortic surgery includes ECG (leads II and V_5), invasive blood pressure monitoring, pulse oximetry, end-tidal CO_2, temperature measurement, esophageal stethoscope insertion, and urine output determination. Invasive blood pressure monitoring is essential to monitor the acute changes in blood pressures that typically accompany aortic surgery. The arterial catheter should be placed in the left radial artery for ascending and transverse arch aneurysms because the repair may involve the brachiocephalic artery. With descending thoracic aneurysms, the optimal placement of the arterial catheter is the right wrist because the operative repair may involve the clamping of the left subclavian artery. (**Ref. 25,** pp. 373–374)

344. **(E)** Carotid artery hemorrhage is one of the most common life-threatening emergencies that arise in patients after carotid endarterectomy. It presents with rapid, large hematoma formation with concomitant airway obstruction. It is recommended in this situation that the wound be opened immediately and before intubation because distorted airway anatomy may complicate intubation. Digital occlusion should be applied to the arteriotomy site to control any ongoing bleeding from the suture lines. The patient should then be transported immediately to the operating room, placed under general anesthesia, and intubated to undergo a formal exploration and repair of the surgical site. (**Ref. 25,** pp. 352–354)

14

Anesthesia for Neurologic Surgery

DIRECTIONS (Questions 345–359): Each of the questions or incomplete statements below is followed by five suggested answers or completions. Select the **one** that is best in each case.

345. Cerebral blood flow can be decreased most effectively by
   A. decrease in MAP
   B. hypoventilation
   C. hyperventilation
   D. sodium nitroprusside
   E. Trendelenburg position

346. The neurosurgeon says the brain is "tight" when he opens the dura for craniotomy for a tumor. A maneuver that would NOT improve this situation is
   A. hyperventilating to $PaCO_2$ of 25 mm Hg
   B. discontinuing inhalation agents and changing to an opioid-barbiturate base anesthesia

C. rotating the head laterally and applying PEEP to improve cerebral blood flow and oxygenation
D. draining spinal fluid through a lumbar catheter
E. ensuring profound muscular relaxation with vecuronium

347. Which of the following statements about evoked potentials is NOT correct?
    A. evoked potentials persist even after the EEG becomes isoelectric
    B. potent inhalational agents increase the amplitude and latency of somatosensory-evoked potentials
    C. temperature, age, and $PaCO_2$ are among several factors that affect evoked potentials
    D. subcortical generators of brain stem auditory evoked potentials are generally more resistant to alteration by anesthetics than are cortical wave forms
    E. the most common use of somatosensory-evoked potential monitoring is for orthopedic correction of scoliosis

348. In an average 70-kg person, the normal CBF is
    A. 75 mL/100 g/min
    B. 1200 mL/min
    C. 50 mL/100 g/min
    D. 120 mL/100 g/min
    E. 250 mL/100 g/min

349. Which of the following drugs is NOT associated with increased intracranial pressure?
    A. ketamine
    B. succinylcholine
    C. sodium nitroprusside
    D. nitroglycerin
    E. esmolol

350. The normal cerebrospinal fluid pressure in the supine position is
    A. 50 mm water
    B. 40 cm water
    C. 110 mm water
    D. 110 cm water
    E. 10 cm water

351. There is correlation among the PaCO$_2$ level, CBF, and ICP:
   A. hyperventilation increases CBF
   B. hyperventilation acts within seconds to decrease CBF and reduce ICP
   C. hyperventilation acts only if PaCO$_2$ level is less than 20 mm Hg
   D. hypoventilation has no effect on CBF if the PaCO$_2$ is less than 50 mm Hg
   E. hyperventilation has no effect if the patient is hypothermic

352. When cerebral autoregulation is disturbed (head injury)
   A. CBF is PaCO$_2$ level dependent
   B. CBF is regulated by adrenergic nervous system
   C. CBF is dependent on arterial blood pressure
   D. CBF is regulated by cerebral metabolic rate
   E. CBF is well preserved

353. All the following drugs have a role in brain protection EXCEPT
   A. barbiturates
   B. propofol
   C. ketamine
   D. etomidate
   E. nimodipine

354. The Glasgow Coma Score is based on
   A. assessment of pupil size
   B. assessment of respiration
   C. assessment of heart rate and rhythm
   D. response to eye opening and motor and verbal response
   E. assessment of tendon reflexes

355. Which of the following statements regarding carotid endarterectomy is NOT correct?
   A. stroke is the most common major complication during and after carotid endarterectomy
   B. myocardial infarction is associated with 25% to 50% of mortality after carotid endarterectomy
   C. the majority of neurologic deficits after carotid endarterectomy are caused by thromboembolism
   D. Major blood loss, up to 1000 mL, is common
   E. Normocarbia is recommended by most of the experts

356. Regarding the effect of nitrous oxide on the brain
    A. N_2O increases CBF more than 60%
    B. N_2O has no effect on ICP increase
    C. N_2O given with volatile agents has no effect on CBF
    D. N_2O decreases CBF
    E. N_2O has no effect on CBF

357. During cerebral aneurysm surgery the surgeon places a temporary vessel clip on the major conductive vessel of the aneurysm. The best protection is usually achieved by
    A. acute hypothermia
    B. induced hypotension
    C. induced hypertension
    D. administration of the barbiturates
    E. increasing $PaCO_2$ level above 40 mm Hg to increase cerebral blood flow

358. Control of ICP during induction includes all of the following EXCEPT
    A. thiopental
    B. narcotic
    C. sodium nitroprusside
    D. nondepolarizing muscle relaxant
    E. short-acting beta blocker

359. The relationship between $PaCO_2$ and cerebral blood flow (CBF) is well known. Therefore, for each mm Hg increase in $PaCO_2$, CBF increases by
    A. 10%
    B. 20%
    C. 2%
    D. 1%
    E. 5%

DIRECTIONS (Questions 360–377): For each of the questions or incomplete statements below, **one** or **more** of the answers given is correct. Select
  A. if only 1, 2, and 3 are correct
  B. if only 1 and 3 are correct
  C. if only 2 and 4 are correct
  D. if only 4 is correct
  E. if all are correct

360. During the sitting position for posterior fossa surgery, early warning signs for venous air embolism include
  1. precordial Doppler monitor changes
  2. ECG changes
  3. transesophageal echocardiograph changes
  4. drop in the end-tidal nitrogen level

361. Enflurane has which of the following characteristics?
  1. it can induce electroencephalographic seizures
  2. it increases CSF production
  3. it produces smaller acute increases in CBF than does halothane
  4. it has no seizure activity if $PaCO_2$ is less than 40 mm Hg

362. The difference between end-tidal CO_2 and the $PaCO_2$ is increased by which of the following conditions?
  1. high cardiac output
  2. low cardiac output
  3. hyperventilation
  4. pulmonary embolism

363. In patients the measurement of cerebral blood flow (CBF), can be performed by
  1. PET scanning
  2. tanscranial Doppler
  3. wash-in/wash-out techniques
  4. EEG power-spectrum analysis

364. During posterior fossa craniotomy, a patient suffers a large venous air embolism:
1. appearance of end-tidal N_2 may be the earliest sign
2. 2-D transesophageal echocardiography shows an unmistakable pattern on its monitor screen
3. end-tidal CO_2 decreases as flow to the lungs is interrupted by the bolus of air
4. pulmonary artery pressure falls precipitously as the right heart suffers acute failure

365. If sodium nitroprusside was infused during cerebral aneurysm surgery, one can expect
1. reflex tachycardia
2. acidosis
3. increase in mixed venous O_2 saturation
4. methemoglobinemia

366. When induced hypothermia is used in neurosurgical procedures
1. the hematocrit drops as temperature decreases
2. blood viscosity increases
3. the platelet count increases when temperature falls below 30°C
4. profound hypothermia has been associated with DIC

367. Mannitol, when used in neurosurgical patients
1. is excluded from the brain by an intact blood–brain barrier (BBB)
2. is filtered by the glomeruli
3. decreases blood viscosity
4. is usually given in a dose of 0.5 to 1 g per kg

368. Adenosine, used for controlled hypotension during cerebral aneurysm surgery
1. increases cardiac index
2. causes tachyphylaxis
3. can be metabolized
4. produces rebound hypertension when discontinued

369. Regional anesthesia used for carotid endarterectomy
1. requires sensory anesthesia of the C_2 to C_4 dermatomes
2. has the advantage of allowing continuous neurologic assessment of the awake patient
3. decreases the requirement for vasoactive drugs
4. has higher incidence of perioperative myocardial infarction

370. During carotid endarterectomy EEG monitoring provides the following information:
1. EEG is a more reliable predictor of intraoperative cerebral ischemia than is neurologic evaluation of the awake patient
2. changes in the EEG correlate closely with the onset and degree of reduction in CBF
3. EEG is most useful when monitored during general anesthesia
4. EEG changes due to intraoperative ischemia include decreases in both frequency and amplitude over the ischemic hemisphere

371. Regarding the control of ICP in patients with brain tumors
1. water restriction that causes dehydration of the brain lowers ICP
2. osmotic diuretics may provide rapid brain dehydration
3. etomidate can acutely reduce ICP
4. steroids in large doses may increase ICP in patients with brain tumors

372. Concerning increased ICP following head trauma, it is true that
1. elevated ICP in the presence of unilateral mass lesion is associated with higher morbidity
2. early after injury, the increased cerebral blood flow (CBF) and cerebral blood volume may lead to ICP elevation
3. hyperventilation is most effective when applied during the hyperemic phase
4. during resuscitation, hyperosmolar glucose solutions are an essential part of the treatment

373. A 58-year-old male is undergoing left carotid endarterectomy. During manipulation of the carotid sinus, the patient develops a bradycardia of 35 bpm and the BP drops to 70/40. You should
   1. administer IV tropine 0.4 to 0.6 mg
   2. ask the surgeon to infiltrate the sinus with lidocaine
   3. inject ephedrine 5 mg IV
   4. massage the ipsilateral carotid artery

374. A 30-year-old man becomes unresponsive after a car accident. In order to declare brain death, the following criteria must be met:
   1. no reflexes
   2. flat EEG (isoelectric at maximum gain)
   3. lack of response to atropine
   4. ICP over 20 mm Hg

375. A patient with a spinal injury above T_4, in the spinal shock phase, will show
   1. hypotension
   2. hypertension
   3. bradycardia
   4. no change in pulse rate

376. Following carotid endarterectomy, the most common complications are
   1. hypertension
   2. hypotension
   3. hematoma formation
   4. decreased ventilation secondary to damage of the carotid body

377. Autonomic hyperreflexia (mass reflex)
   1. is not seen until recovery from spinal shock
   2. is most severe when injury is at T_5 or higher
   3. produces sudden decrease in vascular capacity
   4. may be triggered by mucosal stimulation via pelvic and hypogastric nerves

Anesthesia for Neurologic Surgery

Answers and Discussion

The authors have made every effort to thoroughly verify the answers to the questions that appear on the preceding pages. As in any text, however, some inaccuracies and ambiguities may occur. If in doubt, please consult the indicated reference. When no page number(s) are cited, the reference is to a journal article or to a refresher course lecture that should be read in its entirety.

The Editors

345. (C) Many factors affect cerebral circulation. Positioning may be the most rapid way of initiating change, but hypo- and hypercarbia have the most dramatic and most persistent effects on cerebral vascular resistance. CBF changes 1 to 2 mL/100 g/min for each 1 mm Hg change in $PaCO_2$ around normal $PaCO_2$ values. This response is attenuated below a $PaCO_2$ of 25 mm Hg. Nitroprusside increases CBF, and the Trendelenburg position increases CBV by decreasing venous return. (**Ref. 32,** pp. 624–625)

346. (C) Rotating the head may kink the jugular veins and thus impede venous outflow from the endocranium. This will lead to cerebral congestion. The same result would be achieved by the

Trendelenburg position. PEEP, above a certain level, also impedes venous return from the brain to the thorax and leads not only to decreased cardiac output but also to cerebral congestion. All the other modalities decrease cerebral congestion. (**Ref. 4, #251**)

347. (B) Evoked potentials are computed averages of the brain's responses to repetitive peripheral stimuli. These stimuli may be visual, auditory, or somatosensory. Potent inhalational anesthetic agents decrease the amplitude but increase the latency of the evoked potentials. Evoked potentials do persist when the EEG is isoelectric. (**Ref. 36,** pp. 808–815)

348. (C) In an average, 70-kg person, normal CBF is 50 mL/100 g/min. This represents approximately 15% of the cardiac output. 80% of the flow goes to gray matter and 20% goes to white matter. CBF is regulated by several factors, including CMR (cerebral metabolic rate), $PaCO_2$, PaO_2, autoregulation, neurogenic regulation, and the viscosity of the blood. (**Ref. 32,** p. 622)

349. (E) With the exception of esmolol, all the other drugs increase ICP. Esmolol, a short acting beta-blocker with a half-life of 9 minutes, has also been used successfully to blunt the hypertensive responses that in turn may increase ICP. Na nitroprusside and nitroglycerin cause cerebral vasodilatation and this results in an increase in CBF. Ketamine increases CMR and CBF. Succinylcholine can produce elevation of ICP in lightly anesthetized subjects. This is blocked by deep anesthesia and by defasciculation with metacurine or vecuronium. (**Ref. 14,** pp. 440–441; **Ref. 32,** pp. 627, 633, 641)

350. (C) The intracranial contents consist of three different components: brain, CSF, and blood. The total volume of these factors in the physiologic state is constant; an increase in one is compensated by a decrease in another. In pathologic conditions, the volume of an expanding mass lesion is compensated initially by displacement of equal volumes of blood and CSF out of the cranial cavity. If the space-occupying lesion continues to expand, the compensatory mechanisms will no longer be effective and ICP will increase. Normal CSF pressure in the supine position ranges between 60 and 110 mm of water. (**Ref. 36,** p. 1262)

351. (B) Hyperventilation is of paramount clinical importance when treating a patient with increased intracranial pressure, particularly in the presence of an acute herniation syndrome. Hyperventilation acts within seconds to decrease CBF and thus reduce ICP. After initial decrease, the ICP slowly rises and stabilizes after 3 to 5 hours, usually at a level lower than in the untreated patients. There is little benefit from hyperventilation after 24 to 36 hours. (**Ref. 14,** p. 33)

352. (C) In the acute phase of head injury, cerebral autoregulation is generally impaired. When cerebral autoregulation is disturbed, the CBF is pressure-dependent. This means that arterial hypertension may cause hyperemia and lead to brain swelling (vasogenic edema), which in turn causes an increase in intracranial pressure (ICP). On the other hand, hypotension can lead to cerebral ischemia and may also provoke brain swelling (cytotoxic edema). (**Ref. 6,** #272)

353. (C) All the drugs listed, with the exception of ketamine, have cerebral protective effects. Ketamine is a NMDA antagonist that has produced contradictory findings in a variety of comparable models. Ketamine increases cerebral oxygen consumption and thus cerebral blood flow. It is likely to increase intracranial pressure and should be avoided in patients who already have an elevated ICP. (**Ref. 6,** #172)

354. (D) The Glasgow Coma Score is based on verbal response, on eye opening and on motor response. It awards a maximum of 4 points for eye opening, 6 points for best motor response, and 5 points for best verbal response. Thus, the best possible score is 15. A score of 7 or less usually means that intubation and mechanical hyperventilation are required. The scale has been found to correlate quite well with the injury and also has considerable prognostic significance. (**Ref. 14,** p. 405)

355. (D) During carotid endarterectomy, significant blood loss is uncommon and is usually in the range of 100 to 150 mL. Intravenous access for fluid administration may be limited to one medium-bore (16-gauge) catheter. The main reason blood loss is minimal is the fact that the major arteries are readily accessible to the surgeon and easily clamped, should this become necessary. (**Ref. 36,** p. 1941)

356. (A) The available data indicate unequivocally that N_2O can cause increases in CBF and ICP. When N_2O is added to an already established anesthetic with a volatile anesthetic agent, CBF will increase. In circumstances in which ICP is persistently elevated or the surgical field is persistently tight, N_2O should be viewed as a potential contributing factor. (**Ref. 32,** pp. 639–640)

357. (D) During the period when the major vessel leading to the aneurysm must be clamped, the best protection for the brain is usually provided by barbiturate administration. The main setback in most cases is cardiovascular instability (hypotension). In some centers, therefore, etomidate is being used as an alternative to barbiturates. (**Ref. 14,** pp. 215, 551)

358. (C) For a patient with increased ICP, smooth induction of anesthesia is essential. This is usually accomplished with thiopental 3 to 5 mg/kg, lidocaine 1 mg/kg, and a nondepolarizing muscle relaxant. Esmolol is an example of the short-acting beta blocker that can control BP increases without increasing ICP. Sodium nitroprusside is a potent vasodilator that causes increased CBF and, therefore, increases cerebral blood volume. The end result is an increase of ICP. (**Ref. 32,** p. 1764)

359. (C) CBF varies with $PaCO_2$. Typically, this response is shown to be along a sigmoid curve with inferior and superior plateaus. In the midportion of the curve, the CBF changes by 1.5 to 2 mL/100 g/min for each mm Hg change in $PaCO_2$. It is believed that the responsiveness to CO_2 is driven by changing the extravascular/ interstitial H^+ concentration. (**Ref. 36,** pp. 1608–1609)

360. (B) Precordial Doppler monitoring and the transesophageal echocardiogram provide the earliest warning for venous air embolism (VAE). Precordial Doppler monitoring is much more practical and easier to use than the echocardiogram, which requires continuous visual attention. ECG changes are usually delayed, and end-tidal N_2 actually goes up in the event of VAE. (**Ref. 36,** pp. 1627–1630)

361. **(A)** Enflurane may cause an electroencephalographic seizure pattern, particularly in the presence of hypocapnia (i.e., it requires that the $PaCO_2$ be less than 40 mm Hg). Enflurane-induced seizure activity is associated with substantial increases in CBF and $CMRO_2$. Enflurane, especially in high doses and in the presence of hypocapnia, should be avoided in patients predisposed to seizures and/or with occlusive cerebrovascular disease. (**Ref. 32, p. 638**)

362. **(C)** End-tidal CO_2 monitoring can be thought of as a complement to minute ventilation monitoring. In spontaneously breathing patients subjected to anesthetic-induced respiratory depression, the increased arterial CO_2 tension ($PaCO_2$) is reflected by an increase in end-tidal CO_2 tension (P_{ET} CO_2). P_{ET} CO_2 is normally somewhat lower than $PaCO_2$. This difference is accentuated by general anesthesia and a variety of other abnormal conditions such as chronic obstructive lung disease, low cardiac output, and pulmonary embolism. When pulmonary embolism occurs, a sudden drop in the P_{ET} CO_2 value is diagnostic. Hyperventilation decreases the P_{ET} CO_2 and $PaCO_2$ level simultaneously. (**Ref. 36, p. 77**)

363. **(A)** PET (positron emission tomography) uses radionuclides that emit positrons. The radionuclides are administered by inhalation or by intravenous injection and provide information about local flow. Transcranial Doppler is a measure of the carotid diameter and velocity and provides information about global flow. It is not an invasive technique. In the radioactive tracer washout methods, a diffusible radioactive tracer (e.g., 133 Xe in saline) is injected as a bolus into the internal carotid artery. The rate at which radioactivity disappears from the head can be monitored by using extracranial radiation detectors. The EEG power spectrum analysis is a technique to interpret EEG signals and will not measure CBF. (**Ref. 14, pp. 35–36, 68–69**)

364. **(A)** A large venous air embolus (VAE) will cause the pulmonary artery pressure (PAP) to go up. Increases in PAP can provide a semiquantitative estimate of the volume of VAE. Changes in PAP tend to occur prior to changes in arterial pressure and cardiac output. Following an embolic episode, return of the PAP to-

ward control values can be used as a guide to the recovery from VAE. Changes in PAP and in end-tidal CO_2 tend to occur prior to changes in arterial blood pressure and cardiac output when the total volume and the rate of embolus entrainment are moderate. (**Ref. 32,** p. 1746)

365. **(A)** Methemoglobinemia is a unique systemic side effect associated with a specific local anesthetic agent. It is seen after the administration of large doses of prilocaine. All the other effects can be seen with sodium nitroprusside infusion and toxicity. An additional complication of nitroprusside hypotensive anesthesia is the formation of cyanide. (**Ref. 36,** p. 1250)

366. **(C)** The hematocrit rises as the body temperature falls, and this becomes evident below 30°C. There is a decline in platelet count especially between 25 to 30°C. The CBF falls as the temperature decreases, and this is related to the increased blood viscosity and to the decreased cardiac output (CO). The $CMRO_2$ is reduced and tissue PCO_2 decreases, which also lowers CBF. (**Ref. 32,** pp. 624, 1645–1646)

367. **(E)** Mannitol is prevented from entering the brain by an intact blood–brain barrier (BBB), but if the BBB is damaged in some way, it does permit the passage of mannitol into the brain. Mannitol initially increases blood osmolality and intravascular volume. This potentially dangerous step decreases blood viscosity and, therefore, increases oxygen delivery. Mannitol is an osmotic diuretic eliminated by glomerular filtration. The usual IV dose is 0.5 to 1 g/kg. (**Ref. 14,** pp. 166–167)

368. **(B)** Adenosine has been used for controlled hypotension during cerebral aneurysm surgery. It is characterized by a rapid onset and reversal without any toxicity. There is no tachyphylaxis or rebound hypertension. The cardiac index is increased because of an absence of vasodilatation and the cardiac performance showed no change. Adenosine can be metabolized to uric acid and hypoxanthine but is mainly eliminated by cellular uptake. There is a suggestion that it may blunt cerebral vascular autoregulation. (**Ref. 7,** p. 905)

369. (A) In general, there is no evidence that the risk of regional anesthesia is greater than the risk of general anesthesia. It has been shown that under regional anesthesia there is decreased incidence of perioperative myocardial infarction. Regional anesthesia also allows for the continuous neurologic assessment of the awake patient. This is generally considered to be the most reliable monitor of the adequacy of cerebral perfusion during carotid endarterectomy. (**Ref. 32,** pp. 1710–1711)

370. (C) Changes in the EEG correlate closely with the onset and degree of reduction in cerebral blood flow below a critical threshold in areas of regional cerebral ischemia. EEG changes associated with intraoperative ischemia include decreases in both frequency and amplitude over the ischemic hemisphere. Modern advances in EEG signal processing, such as computer-assisted power spectrum analysis, have promoted increasing use of intraoperative EEG monitoring as a method of detecting acute, cross–clamp-related cerebral ischemia during carotid endarterectomy. (**Ref. 32,** p. 1711)

371. (A) Dehydration of the brain lowers ICP. Water intake limited to about one-third to one-half of daily fluid requirements may accomplish this reduction over a period of several days. More rapid dehydration of the brain can be obtained by employing diuretic agents. Etomidate decreases CBF, and this leads to a reduction of the ICP. In patients with cerebral edema and increased ICP secondary to brain tumor, very large doses of steroids may decrease ICP and improve neurologic function. (**Ref. 32,** pp. 1754–1759)

372. (A) Studies have shown that hyperglycemia existing before an ischemic or hypoxic event enhances ischemic damage. Thus, following head injury, it would seem appropriate to avoid sugar-containing solutions and maintain systemic blood pressure with colloid infusions. (**Ref. 14,** pp. 424–428)

373. (A) Intraoperative manipulation of the carotid sinus may cause bradycardia, hypotension, and reduction in flow across the stenotic area. The reflex arc involves the glossopharyngeal nerve (IX), the medulla, and the vagus nerve (X). The reflex can be blocked by infiltrating the carotid sinus with lidocaine or by the intravenous administration of 0.4 to 0.6 mg of atropine. Sometimes, in spite of the atropine injection, the blood pressure may stay low. In that case, ephedrine 5 to 10 mg or isoproterenol (1 mg in 500 mL solution) may be given by IV infusion. (**Ref. 14, pp. 187–189**)

374. (A) The diagnosis of brain death requires a combination of clinical findings that include unresponsive coma, apnea, unreactive, dilated pupils, and absent brain stem reflexes. Laboratory studies should show an isoelectric EEG and the absence of cerebral blood flow. Persistence of clinical findings and isoelectric EEG for more than 3 hours should confirm the diagnosis. (**Ref. 14, p. 573**)

375. (B) The extent of these changes is a function of the level of the cord injury. Patients with injuries at or above the T_4 level, will develop hypotension and bradycardia during the spinal shock phase. The observed bradycardia may be due to unopposed vagal tone, secondary to loss of the cardiac accelerator fibers (T_1–T_4). But many feel that the Bainbridge reflex triggered by a fall in right atrial and central venous pressures is also an important contributing factor to the bradycardia seen with lesions below T_4 levels. This phase of the spinal shock may last days to weeks. (**Ref. 36, pp. 276–280**)

376. (A) Hypertension and hypotension are frequent complications of carotid endarterectomy. The mechanism of acute hypertension is thought to involve denervation of the carotid sinus during mobilization of the carotid bifurcation, with resultant loss of the tonic baroreceptor activity. Hypotension is usually associated with bradycardia, and the usual cause of this problem is plaque removal from the region of the carotid baroreceptors. This exposes these pressure receptors to higher pressure, increasing their discharge to the medulla of the brain and resulting in vagally induced bradycardia and hypotension. The baroreceptors will adjust to the new pressure gradually over several hours. Ventilation in one-sided carotid endarterectomy is usually unaffected. But particular attention should be paid to patients who have had bilateral carotid endarterectomy performed within 12 months and who may have sustained damage to their carotid body. (**Ref. 32, p. 1728**)

377. **(E)** 85% of the patients with T_6 or higher injury have autonomic hyperreflexia. It is typically seen after distention of the bladder or bowel but may happen even with a milder stimulus. Hypertension can be very severe—severe enough to cause intracranial and retinal hemorrhages. For this reason autonomic hyperreflexia should be prevented whenever possible and should be treated as a medical emergency if it does occur. (**Ref. 36,** p. 260)

15

Pain Management

DIRECTIONS (Questions 378–393): Each of the questions or incomplete statements below is followed by five suggested answers or completions. Select the **one** that is best in each case.

378. A 59-year-old female has a history of chronic low back pain due to osteoarthritis. The most appropriate treatment is
   A. epidural steroid injection
   B. spinal traction and physical therapy
   C. NSAID (nonsteroidal anti-inflammatory drugs)
   D. tricyclic antidepressants
   E. surgical intervention with laminectomy

379. Confirmation of the diagnosis of peripheral neuropathy is best achieved by using
   A. diagnostic nerve block
   B. thermography
   C. EMG
   D. nerve conduction studies
   E. sweat test

380. Regarding the treatment of trigeminal neuralgia, correct statements include all of the following EXCEPT
   A. treatment directed peripherally is generally not successful
   B. carbamazepine is the standard medical therapy
   C. radio frequency lesioning of the ganglion may result in the relief of symptoms
   D. stellate ganglion block on the affected side is very effective in stopping paroxysmal pain
   E. glycerol injections into the trigeminal ganglion have been useful in selected patients

381. The signs of causalgia include all of the following EXCEPT
   A. superficial burning pain
   B. hyperpathia
   C. pain usually paroxysmal in nature
   D. atrophic changes
   E. autonomic dysfunction

382. The following statements regarding intraspinal opioids are all correct EXCEPT
   A. substance P release is known to be inhibited by morphine
   B. intraspinal opioids play their greatest role at the level of the substantia gelatinosa of the dorsal horn of the spinal cord
   C. morphine binds primarily to the μ receptor
   D. the μ receptor is most dominant in producing analgesia
   E. the elimination half-life for morphine in CSF is approximately 12 hours

383. Opioids, when used epidurally, are least likely to produce
   A. orthostatic hypotension secondary to sympathetic block
   B. respiratory depression
   C. opioid withdrawal syndrome
   D. nausea and vomiting
   E. urinary retention

384. For postoperative pain relief, an intercostal block should be performed
   A. paravertebrally
   B. at the costal angle

C. at the posterior axillary line
D. at the midaxillary line
E. at the anterior axillary line

385. Meralgia paresthetica is thought to be due to compression of which of the following nerves?
    A. obturator
    B. saphenous
    C. lateral femoral cutaneous
    D. pudendal
    E. sural

386. Which of the following observations regarding the myofascial pain syndrome are NOT correct?
    A. pain usually is shooting in nature
    B. treatment may include injection with local anesthetics into the trigger points
    C. EMG is positive in 70% of the cases
    D. it can occur spontaneously
    E. depression in chronic cases is common

387. The clinical indications for stellate ganglion block with a local anesthetic include all EXCEPT
    A. postembolectomy spasm
    B. causalgia of the arm
    C. phantom limb pain
    D. Sudeck's atrophy
    E. multiple sclerosis

388. The substantia gelatinosa
    A. is in the cortex of the brain
    B. is located in the lateral columns
    C. has the highest concentration of opioid receptors in the spinal cord
    D. is a part of the posterior column
    E. is located in the cauda equina of the spinal cord

389. The following statements regarding the stellate ganglion are all correct EXCEPT
    A. at the level of the stellate ganglia, the vertebral artery lies anterior to them
    B. the stellate ganglion supplies sympathetic innervation to the upper extremity
    C. it lies at the level of the fifth cervical vertebra
    D. it is the fusion of the inferior cervical and first thoracic ganglia
    E. the apex of the lung is closer on the right than the left

390. All the following features of the trigeminal neuralgia (tic douloureux) are correct EXCEPT
    A. pain is intermittent
    B. it is usually unilateral
    C. there are autonomic changes
    D. the most common cause is vascular compression of a nerve in the subarachnoid space
    E. the age of onset is often over 50 years old

391. Which of the following painful conditions will NOT benefit from a lumbar sympathetic block?
    A. reflex sympathetic dystrophy of the lower extremity
    B. periphery vascular insufficiency
    C. chronic pancreatitis
    D. acute herpes zoster
    E. pain from cancer of the gastrointestinal track distal to the transverse colon

392. The sympathetic nerve supply to the arm is derived from
    A. C_5–C_8
    B. C_5–T_1
    C. C_4–T_2
    D. T_2–T_9
    E. T_1–T_4

393. The stellate ganglion block results in the interruption of the following nerve fiber(s):
   A. B fibers
   B. C fibers
   C. B and C fibers
   D. A delta fibers
   E. B and A delta fibers

DIRECTIONS (Questions 394–417): For each of the questions or incomplete answers below, **one** or **more** of the answers or completions are correct. Select
   A. if only 1, 2, and 3 are correct
   B. if only 1 and 3 are correct
   C. if only 2 and 4 are correct
   D. if only 4 is correct
   E. if all are correct

---

394. In making the diagnosis of advanced reflex sympathetic dystrophy (RSD)
   1. the plain x-ray film shows patchy osteoporosis
   2. skin temperature measured from the pulp of the digits of the upper and lower extremities provides a crude estimate of the severity of the disorder
   3. three-phase radionuclide bone scanning shows great diagnostic sensitivity
   4. EMG is usually positive

395. Four weeks prior to his admission, a 36-year-old male develops low back pain after lifting heavy boxes. The pain radiates along the S_1 dermatome. You would
   1. administer epidural steroid injection (ESI)
   2. obtain neurosurgical consent
   3. start on oral NSAID (nonsteroidal anti-inflammatory drugs)
   4. prescribe bed rest for 10 days, oral pain medication, and daily physical therapy

396. Celiac plexus block can alleviate pain originating from the following organs:
1. liver
2. pancreas
3. stomach
4. bladder

397. The successful sympathetic block can be evaluated with
1. sweat test
2. psychogalvanic response (PGR)
3. thermography
4. plethysmography

398. A 76-year-old female complains of severe pain in the left thoracic region secondary to postherpetic neuralgia. You would recommend
1. epidural steroid injection
2. tricyclic antidepressants
3. phenytoin
4. rhizotomy

399. When a celiac plexus block is performed with alcohol to control the pain secondary to carcinoma of the pancreas, the complications may include
1. orthostatic hypotension
2. puncture of the bladder
3. pneumothorax
4. Horner's syndrome

400. A 30-year-old woman complained of severe diffuse burning pain in the right hand and forearm that started 3 months ago following blunt trauma. Measurement of skin temperature showed that the right hand was 5 degrees colder than the left hand. You would recommend
1. aggressive physical therapy
2. a stellate ganglion block on the affected side
3. an intravenous regional sympathetic block using reserpine
4. oral corticosteroids and tricyclic antidepressants

401. A 35-year-old male with the diagnosis of early RSD of the right hand, receives a right stellate ganglion block. Following the block, the patient develops right-sided Horner's syndrome but reports no pain relief. Your conclusion would be
1. patient did not have sympathetic block to upper extremity
2. the diagnosis is incorrect
3. there was a failure to anesthetize nerve of Kuntz
4. there was a technical failure in performing of stellate ganglion block

402. Which of the following statement(s) about sympathetically maintained pain (SMP) is (are) true?
1. burning pain is a common complaint
2. the diagnosis can usually be made clinically by history and associated physical findings
3. causalgia and reflex sympathetic dystrophy (RSD) are the most common SMP syndromes
4. local anesthesia sympathetic block is very effective in the early phase

403. Factors that increase the incidence of respiratory depression from epidural narcotics include
1. dural puncture
2. age greater than 55
3. concomitant administration of parenteral opioids
4. using a mixture of opioids and local anesthetics

404. Correct statements regarding postherpetic neuralgia include
1. the etiology is unclear
2. sympathetic blocks are effective during early phase
3. tricyclic antidepressants are effective in some cases
4. anticonvulsants are contraindicated since they may aggravate the symptoms

405. A 30-year-old male received a neurolytic lumbar sympathetic block for reflex sympathetic dystrophy of the right foot. Complications include
1. neuritis
2. chronic orthostatic hypotension
3. anesthesia dolorosa
4. thrombophlebitis

406. Epidural blockade, administered with local anesthetics, has the following advantages over epidural opioids:
1. less interference with intestinal motility
2. less systemic toxic effects, like nausea and pruritus
3. better protection against metabolic and endocrine responses to surgical trauma
4. lower incidence of urinary retention

407. When absolute alcohol is used for a subarachnoid block to alleviate cancer pain
1. the total dose should not exceed 1.5 mL
2. the likelihood of good results is about 50%
3. the patient is placed in a lateral position with the affected side up
4. the injection time should be more than 2 min

408. Correct statements regarding central pain include
1. the pain usually involves half of the whole body
2. the lesion is frequently in the thalamus
3. may be relieved by medications such as the phenothiazines and tricyclic antidepressants
4. intrathecal opioids are very effective in eliminating the pain

409. A 60-year-old male has the diagnosis of bladder cancer. The patient complains of severe pelvic pain. You are consulted for pain control and recommend
1. celiac plexus block
2. hypogastric plexus block
3. rhizotomy of the sacral nerve roots
4. epidural catheter implantation for continuous opioid administration

410. Statements regarding the whiplash syndrome include
1. the term whiplash describes an abrupt hyperextension injury of the neck
2. usually the cervical flexor muscles and specifically the sternocleidomastoid muscle are affected
3. treatment is conservative but in selected cases nerve blocks may help
4. opioids play major role in the control of the spastic pain

411. The most common characteristics of acute lumbar radiculopathy are
1. the dermatomal distribution of the pain
2. epidural steroid injections are effective in only 20% of the cases
3. the tendon reflexes are diminished
4. anticonvulsants are effective in controlling the pain

412. The most common findings in chronic pancreatitis are
1. 100% of patients suffer from chronic abdominal pain
2. a lumbar sympathetic block is the best choice to control the pain
3. narcotic addiction is common
4. 20% of patients have history of alcoholism

413. The clinical profile of the cluster headaches syndrome is characterized by
1. unilateral pain
2. primarily female population
3. accompanying autonomic phenomena
4. a population primarily 60 years old and over

414. Different types of pain are known to be transmitted by different types of nerve fibers. Thus
1. visceral pain is carried mostly by unmyelinated C fibers
2. B fibers are responsible for transmission of the fast pain
3. somatic pain is transmitted by the large myelinated A fibers
4. sympathetically mediated pain is carried by C fibers

415. Horner's syndrome results if the cervical sympathetic fibers (stellate ganglion) are successfully blocked. The clinical signs of Horner's syndrome include
1. ptosis on affected side
2. miosis on affected side
3. enophthalmos on affected side
4. mydriasis on affected side

416. A 25-year-old female with a 4-month history of reflex sympathetic dystrophy of the left hand receives an intravenous regional sympathetic block with guanethidine
1. guanethidine displaces norepinephrine from the presynaptic vesicles and inhibits its reuptake
2. if guanethidine is not available, reserpine may be used for the intravenous regional block
3. guanethidine should not be administered to patients taking MAO inhibitors
4. the tourniquet should be kept inflated for at least 60 min

417. Subarachnoid alcohol blockade offers great pain relief in selected patients with advanced cancer.
1. the usual concentration of alcohol is 95% (absolute)
2. the major complications include neuritis and motor weakness
3. during the injection, the patient is at a 45° angle with the painful side uppermost
4. 95% alcohol is a hyperbaric solution

Pain Management

Answers and Discussion

The authors have made every effort to thoroughly verify the answers to the questions that appear on the preceding pages. As in any text, however, some inaccuracies and ambiguities may occur. If in doubt, please consult the indicated reference. When no page number(s) are cited, the reference is to a journal arricle or to a refresher course lecture that should be read in its entirety.

The Editors

378. **(C)** Osteoarthritis is the most common indication for which an NSAID is prescribed. Epidural steroid injections can be helpful if there is a sign of nerve root irritation or involvement. Tricyclic antidepressants have a major role in the treatment of the chronic pain syndromes, especially when they are accompanied by depression. (**Ref. 45,** pp. 170–171)

379. **(D)** Neuropathy is a disturbance of function or a pathologic change in the nerves. It may affect a single nerve or several. The clinical features may include pain, muscle atrophy, cramps, and loss of tendon reflexes. Confirmation of the diagnosis of peripheral neuropathy is best achieved through nerve conduction studies. EMG is usually used to differentiate a myopathy from a peripheral neuropathy. (**Ref. 45,** p. 295)

380. **(D)** According to some neurosurgeons, the cause of this disease is the impinging of blood vessels on the nerve in the region of the ganglion. It is important to recognize that in some patients, especially those younger than 40 years of age, symptoms of trigeminal neuralgia may indicate an underlying disease process, such as multiple sclerosis or a space-occupying lesion at the cerebellopontine angle. Treatment of the primary trigeminal neuralgia initially is medical. Carbamazepine is effective in some cases. Radio frequency lesioning of the ganglion or glycerol injections into the trigeminal ganglion have been useful in selected cases. Stellate ganglion blocks are not an effective way to treat trigeminal neuralgia since the pathophysiology is most likely to be central and not sympathetically mediated. (**Ref. 45,** p. 104)

381. **(C)** The major signs of causalgia may include pain that is described as superficial, burning, deep crushing, or stabbing pain. It is usually secondary to a gunshot wound. There are findings of autonomic dysfunction. Hyperpathia and allodynia accompany some dystrophic changes (brittle nails, osteoporosis). Paroxysmal pain is usually characteristic of painful conditions like trigeminal neuralgia. (**Ref. 45,** pp. 219–220; **Ref. 1,** pp. 178–180)

382. **(E)** Evidence indicates that intraspinal opiates play their greatest role at the level of the substantia gelatinosa of the dorsal horn of the spinal cord. There are several naturally occurring peptides that are known to affect pain. Substance P has been identified at the peripheral nerve endings in the dorsal root ganglia and centrally. Its release is known to be inhibited by morphine. Morphine is much less lipid soluble and, therefore, it is slow to diffuse through the dura, slow to bind to receptor sites, and slow to exit. The elimination half-life of morphine in CSF is approximately 2 hours (range 60 to 258 minutes). (**Ref. 45,** pp. 363–365)

383. **(A)** An epidural or intrathecal injection of morphine clearly causes more complete pain relief than systemic injection and may decrease postoperative morbidity and mortality in certain patient populations. In patients receiving epidural opioid after previous long-term treatment with parenteral opioids, the amount of opioid reaching the tolerant brain may not be sufficient to prevent a withdrawal response if opioid administration by other routes is suddenly discontinued when pain relief is obtained. Respiratory depression secondary to epidural morphine administration ranges between 0.25% and 0.4%. Certain risk factors, which include age over 65, high doses of morphine, concomitant parenteral administration of narcotics and sedatives, may increase the possibility of respiratory depression. Nausea is a more frequent side effect in obstetric patients. Urinary retention occurs most often in young male patients. Orthostatic hypotension due to sympathetic blockade with epidural opioids is unusual, since the opioids do not cause neural blockade. (**Ref. 11,** pp. 993–996; **Ref. 36,** pp. 1429–1431)

384. (D) Intercostal nerve block of the appropriate nerves can give excellent pain relief. It was recommended that the intercostal nerves be blocked close to the angle of the rib. Recent studies have shown that injections into the intercostal space travel several centimeters in either direction from the tip of the needle. Good blocks are therefore obtainable in the midaxillary line and with much less discomfort to the patient. (**Ref. 11,** p. 17)

385. (C) The lateral cutaneous nerve of the thigh is a purely sensory nerve formed from the posterior divisions of L_2 and L_3. It innervates the outer lateral aspect of the thigh. Symptoms include burning pain and dysesthesias along the lateral aspect of the thigh. The most common site of lateral femoral cutaneous nerve entrapment appears to be where the nerve passes from the pelvis into the thigh. Pressure from belts or girdles can be the precipitating cause. (**Ref. 45,** p. 185)

386. (C) The myofascial pain syndrome (MPS) is a condition characterized by aching pain arising from muscles and associated with stiffness. It can occur spontaneously or after an injury to the muscular structure. The cause of MPS is unknown. The diagnosis is established by demonstrating the painful trigger points that, when stimulated by pressure, produce radiating pain. There is no diagnostic test for MPS, and the EMG is usually normal. (**Ref. 45,** pp. 259–263; **Ref. 1,** pp. 99–104)

387. (E) The clinical indications for a stellate ganglion block include a long list of conditions. Most of the indications are based largely on anecdotal case reports so that an initial diagnostic blockade should always be accompanied by individual assessment. Multiple sclerosis is a neurologic disease that mainly involves the spinal cord and has no specific treatment. (**Ref. 11,** p. 480)

388. **(C)** The complex synaptic structures of the substantia gelatinosa include terminals of the primary afferent fibers, terminals of the local axons and dendrites, and terminals of the brain stem neurons that descend to all levels of the cord. The substantia gelatinosa also has the highest concentration of opioid receptors. It is located in the dorsal horn area of the spinal cord. (**Ref. 45,** p. 17)

389. **(C)** In most individuals the inferior cervical ganglion is fused to the first thoracic ganglion, forming the stellate ganglion. It usually lies in front of the neck of the first rib and extends to the interspace between C_7 and T_1. At the level of the stellate ganglia, the vertebral artery lies anterior. The stellate ganglion supplies sympathetic innervation to the upper extremity through the gray communicating rami of C_7, C_8, T_1 and occasionally of C_5 and C_6. (**Ref. 36,** pp. 1367–1368)

390. **(C)** Trigeminal neuralgia is a disease of the elderly, but occurs occasionally in young adults as well. The peak incidence is between ages 50 and 70. Pain is unilateral, like an electric shock, and stabbing in nature. There are pain-free intervals between attacks, and there are no autonomic changes. (**Ref. 9,** pp. 676–679)

391. **(C)** Lumbar sympathetic blocks have been used extensively in the treatment of sympathetically mediated pain. Peripheral vascular insufficiency continues to be the major indication for sympathetic blockade. Patients with acute herpes zoster and, possibly, postherpetic neuralgia can also benefit from lumbar sympathetic blockade. Improved circulation to the vasa-nervosum and peripheral structures can decrease inflammation and prevent further neuronal damage caused by the virus. The pancreas is innervated by the celiac plexus, and therefore pain control in chronic pancreatitis requires celiac plexus blockade. (**Ref. 36,** pp. 1381–1382; **Ref. 11,** pp. 491–492)

392. **(D)** The preganglionic sympathetic outflow to the upper extremity is derived from T_2–T_3, and these fibers synapse with postganglionic fibers in the stellate ganglion. The brachial plexus supplies

all the motor and sensory functions of the arm. The brachial plexus is formed from the anterior primary rami of the fifth, sixth, seventh, and eighth cervical and first thoracic nerves, and frequently receives some contributing branches from the fourth cervical and second thoracic nerve. (**Ref. 36,** p. 1367; **Ref. 11,** p. 388)

393. **(C)** The stellate ganglion block results in the interruption of conduction along the preganglionic, thinly myelinated B fibers and of the postganglionic, unmyelinated C fibers. (**Ref. 11,** p. 462)

394. **(A)** In the advanced stages of RSD, patchy osteoporosis is observed and three-phase bone scanning has been shown to be one of the most sensitive tests available. EMG and nerve conduction studies are most useful in distinguishing between a myopathic and a neurogenic origin of peripheral neuromuscular pathology. (**Ref. 45,** pp. 59, 220)

395. **(B)** In acute low back pain, without neurologic or sensory deficit but with radicular pain, conservative therapy is always desirable. This may include ESI, 50 mg triamcinolone or placing 80 mg of methylprednisolone as close as possible to the level of nerve root irritation. A short bed rest of 2 to 3 days with oral aspirin or NSAID is an alternative.

    Neurosurgical consultation should be obtained if there are signs of motor, sensory, or reflex changes. Pain alone is not an indication for surgery. Prolonged bed rest is known to cause muscle weakness and decalcification of the bones. It is not a part of a proper treatment. (**Ref. 1,** pp. 109–114)

396. **(A)** The celiac plexus lies anterior to the aorta in the epigastrium. It is also located just anterior to the crus of the diaphragm. The plexus extends for several centimeters in front of the aorta and laterally around the aorta. Postganglionic nerves from these ganglia innervate all the abdominal viscera with the exception of part of the transverse colon, left colon, rectum, and pelvic viscera. Any pain originating from the visceral structures innervated by the celiac plexus can be alleviated by blockade of this plexus. The bladder is innervated by the inferior mesenteric ganglion. (**Ref. 36,** pp. 1373–1374)

397. **(E)** Evidence of sympathetic blockade of the upper extremity includes visible engorgement of the veins of the extremity, psychogalvanic reflex (PGR), thermography, plethysmography, and sweat test. A rise in skin temperature also occurs. (**Ref. 36, p. 1371**)

398. **(A)** Epidural steroid injections, tricyclic antidepressants, and phenytoin (anticonvulsant) have been used with some success and are considered to be frontline therapeutic options. Surgery (rhizotomy) is the last resort for the treatment of severe intractable postherpetic pain. It is not always successful and generally has poor results. (**Ref. 45, pp. 286–291**)

399. **(B)** The celiac plexus is located in front of the body of L_1, and therefore puncture of the liver, spleen, kidney, pancreas, or ureter is possible. The bladder is located in the pelvis and far away from the block area. Orthostatic hypotension is not uncommon, and it is a result of the sympathetic block. Horner's syndrome is one of the signs of the successful stellate ganglion block. Since the aorta and the inferior vena cava are adjacent to the celiac plexus, puncture of these structures is also possible. (**Ref. 45, pp. 521–523**)

400. **(E)** When a patient is diagnosed to have early reflex sympathetic dystrophy (RSD), the treatment of choice is sympathetic block and physiotherapy. Other forms of therapy that have been tried with some success and that may be used are IV regional sympathetic block using guanethidine, reserpine, or bretylium, and oral sympatholytic agents such as prazosin, propranolol, corticosteroids, and tricyclic antidepressants. In some centers, transcutaneous electric stimulation is also used. (**Ref. 45, pp. 227–228**)

401. **(B)** The appearance of Horner's syndrome indicates only the interruption of the sympathetic supply to the head and neck. Unless it is accompanied by other signs of successful sympathetic blockade, it does not indicate a sympathetic block of the upper extremity. The patient may have a very impressive Horner's syndrome but minimal or no sympathetic interruption to the upper extremity. This can happen when the volume of the local anesthetic is too small, or when the patient stays supine instead of having the head and neck elevated after the block. In approximately 10% to

20% of the population, the nerve of Kuntz is responsible for the sympathetic innervation to the upper extremity. Fibers in the nerve of Kuntz may originate from the upper thoracic segments and innervate the upper extremity without passing through the stellate ganglia. (**Ref. 45,** pp. 227–228)

402. (E) The term sympathetically maintained pain (SMP) refers to syndromes that characterize those effects on the body (usually on an extremity) that are mediated by sympathetic nervous system dysfunction after trauma, or that are caused by visceral or CNS disease. Reflex sympathetic dystrophy (RSD) and causalgia are the two most common forms of SMP. In RSD, a history of specific nerve injury is not always elicited. In causalgia, there is always at least partial nerve damage. (**Ref. 9,** pp. 220–243)

403. (A) Dural puncture allows the transfer of opioid from the epidural to subarachnoid space. This situation, especially with hydrophilic drugs such as morphine sulfate, can cause significant respiratory depression. Concomitant systemic administration of opioids is the largest risk factor for respiratory depression, since epidural opioids and parenteral opioids may reach the fourth ventricle at the same time and cause respiratory depression. It has been shown that age over 55 years is a predisposing factor for respiratory depression. Addition of a local anesthetic will not increase the risk of respiratory depression unless a very large volume is used. (**Ref. 36,** pp. 1429–1430)

404. (B) Somatic or sympathetic nerve blocks should be attempted early after the onset of the postherpetic neuralgia. Epidural steroids also show some beneficial effects. Anticonvulsants such as phenytoin and valproic acid are useful agents and are included in the treatment of postherpetic neuralgia. The etiology is still unclear in spite of tremendous research efforts. (**Ref. 45,** pp. 287–292)

405. (B) Neuritis has been reported to have an incidence of about 10%. Anesthesia dolorosa is a distressing condition of numbness that is presently poorly understood. Other complications of the neurolytic blocks include sloughing of the skin and prolonged motor paralysis. Patients may experience temporary orthostatic hypotension, but in the average, healthy person, compensation for the regional vasodilatation occurs. Thrombophlebitis is not a problem because blood flow usually improves. (**Ref. 1,** pp. 292–293; **Ref. 11,** pp. 730–731)

406. (A) Epidural analgesia with a local anesthetic is associated with significantly earlier return of bowel motility than when systemic opioids are used for postoperative pain control. It seems that epidural local anesthetics provide for better bowel motility than do epidural opioids. Urinary retention is a potential problem with both techniques. Nausea and pruritus are known side effects of the opioids. Regional blockade with local anesthetics to prevent stress responses to surgical trauma is shown to be more effective than opioids. (**Ref. 5,** #275)

407. (E) To limit the spread of alcohol in the subarachnoid space to the affected segments, the volume of solution injected should be less than 1.5 mL, and the rate of injection should be more than 2 min. If the area involved is relatively extensive, multiple level injections of small volumes (0.5 mL not to exceed a total of 1.5 mL) are preferable to a single, larger injection. To treat bilateral pain, the injection can be made with the patient prone and flexed and with the affected segments uppermost over the break in the operating table. (**Ref. 11,** pp. 1056–1057)

408. (A) Dejerine and Roussy originally described central pain in a group of the patients with strokes that was characterized by diffuse, unilateral burning pain that usually affected half of the whole body. Spinal cord injuries are also responsible for a number of central pain cases. Therapy usually involves centrally acting medications such as phenothiazines and tricyclic antidepressants. These patients are sometimes helped by carbamazepine and diphenylhydantoin. Other treatment options include dorsal cord stimulation and deep brain stimulation. Opioids are not effective in this type of pain syndrome. (**Ref. 45,** pp. 311–312; **Ref. 11,** p. 759)

409. (C) The cervical plexus block is an effective treatment option for upper abdominal visceral pain. Hypogastric plexus blockade at L_5–S_1 level can also be an effective treatment for pain associated with pelvic visceral cancers (bladder). The indications for rhizotomy for cancer pain seem to be limited to individual nerve roots in the thoracic and cervical region. Currently, epidural or intraspinal catheter implantation for opioid and/or low concentration local anesthetic administration is becoming a very popular treatment option for cancer pain. (**Ref. 45,** pp. 252–253; **Ref. 11,** pp. 1004–1006)

410. (A) The initial treatment is conservative. Soft cervical collar, analgesics, and bed rest with gradual increase in activity for the first 1 to 2 weeks. Transcutaneous electrical nerve stimulation (TENS) may be helpful. There is no place for opioids in the treatment of this type of pain condition. On the other hand, especially in chronic cases, nerve blocks may provide great relief. (**Ref. 45,** pp. 112–114)

411. (B) The signs and symptoms of acute lumbar radiculopathy may include low back pain radiating to the lower extremity, usually dermatomal in distribution. The pain may be of a shooting or electrical quality. There are diminished sensations in the affected dermatome and diminished reflexes. Pain on straight leg raising can be very dramatic. Laboratory studies may show positive EMG, MRI, and CT scan results. If pain has been present for less than six months, about 60% of the patients may achieve good and lasting pain relief from epidural steroid injections. Anticonvulsants have been used for chronic cases and have occasionally been effective. (**Ref. 1,** pp. 108–115)

412. (B) Pain is the central feature of chronic pancreatitis. The pain can vary in intensity but never subsides completely and frequently radiates to the back. Most dramatic pain relief can be obtained by performing a celiac plexus block with a local anesthetic or 70% alcohol. In most instances, the medical management of chronic pancreatic pain relies on the use of narcotic analgesics that in the long run leads to physical dependence. The cause of chronic pancreatitis in 80% to 90% of the patients is chronic alcoholism. (**Ref. 9,** pp. 1225–1226)

413. (B) The clinical profile of the cluster headache syndrome is characterized by unilateral pain, by the temporal patterns of the attacks, and by the accompanying autonomic phenomena. Males are affected about 5 to 9 times as often as females. Cluster headaches are rarely encountered in patients above the age of 60. (**Ref. 9,** pp. 716–717)

414. (B) The nerve fibers have been divided into three major groups. The myelinated, somatic nerves are called A fibers. The thinnest A fibers, the delta group, perform fast pain transmissions, sense temperature, and signal tissue damage. The thinly myelinated B fibers are preganglionic autonomic axons that innervate vascular smooth muscle and are responsible for the transmissions of sympathetically mediated pain. C fibers are nonmyelinated and thinner than the myelinated fibers. C fibers subserve slow pain and temperature transmission and postganglionic autonomic functions. (**Ref. 11,** p. 35)

415. (A) Horner's syndrome appears if the cervical sympathetic fibers are successfully blocked. Signs of Horner's syndrome are ptosis (dropping of the upper eyelid), miosis (small pupil), enophthalmos (sunken eyeball), and anhidrosis (lack of sweating). All these signs appear on the same side as the block. (**Ref. 11,** p. 480)

416. (A) When local anesthetic blocks of the sympathetic chain fail to improve sympathetically maintained pain (SMP) in an extremity, an intravenous regional block with sympatholytic drugs (guanethidine and reserpine) is an appropriate alternative. Guanethidine's site of action is the postganglionic neuron at the neuroeffector junction. It displaces norepinephrine from presynaptic vesicles and inhibits its reuptake. Reserpine may have a mechanism of action similar to that of guanethidine. Tourniquet time of 20 to 30 min is sufficient to fix the guanethidine and to prevent its release into the systemic circulation. (**Ref. 36,** pp. 1385–1387)

417. (A) Intrathecal neurolysis with alcohol is appropriate for cancer patients with a short life expectancy and well localized pain. The positioning of the patient is of paramount importance if alcohol, a hypobaric solution, is used for intrathecal injection. The patient is positioned at a 45° angle, with the painful side uppermost. Neuritis and motor weakness are the two major disadvantages of alcohol blockade. (**Ref. 36,** pp. 1407–1412)

16
Anesthesia for Urological Surgery

DIRECTIONS (Questions 418–429): For each of the questions or incomplete answers below, **one** or **more** of the answers or completions are correct. Select
- **A.** if only 1, 2, and 3 are correct
- **B.** if only 1 and 3 are correct
- **C.** if only 2 and 4 are correct
- **D.** if only 4 is correct
- **E.** if all are correct

---

418. Complication(s) associated with the absorption of irrigation fluid during transurethral resection (TURP) of the prostate include
1. seizures
2. hypothermia
3. transient blindness
4. hypernatremia

242 / 16: Anesthesia for Urological Surgery

419. The following fluid(s) is (are) suitable for irrigation in transurethral resection of the prostate
    1. sorbitol 2.7% and mannitol 0.54%
    2. normal saline
    3. glycine 1.5%
    4. sterile water

420. Which of the following nondepolarizing muscle relaxants is (are) suitable for intraoperative use in a patient with end-stage renal disease?
    1. pancuronium
    2. atracurium
    3. gallamine
    4. vecuronium

421. Abnormalities associated with renal cell carcinoma include
    1. hypercalcemia
    2. hypertension
    3. Cushing's syndrome
    4. hyperthyroidism

422. The following condition(s) will decrease the induction dose of thiopental
    1. chronic renal failure
    2. advanced age
    3. cirrhosis
    4. alkalosis

423. Laboratory values associated with prerenal oliguria include
    1. urine osmolality > 500 mOsm/L
    2. urine Na^+ < 20
    3. urine CR/plasma CR < 20
    4. fractional excretion of Na^+ > 2

424. Possible cause(s) of perioperative bleeding from transurethral resection of the prostate (TURP) include
    1. dilutional thrombocytopenia
    2. disseminated intravascular coagulation
    3. irritation of prostatic tissue from the bladder catheter
    4. poor platelet function

425. The ECG manifestations of hyperkalemia include
  1. peaked T waves
  2. ST segment depression
  3. widening of the QRS complex
  4. dysrhythmias

426. In a routine urinalysis, the following finding(s) may be normal
  1. pH 5.0
  2. trace proteinuria
  3. no heme
  4. 1+ glucose

427. Which of the following are associated with perioperative renal failure?
  1. aortic cross-clamping
  2. aminoglycosides
  3. cardiopulmonary bypass
  4. intravascular volume contraction

428. Which of the following inhalational anesthetic agent(s) should be avoided in patients with renal insufficiency?
  1. isoflurane
  2. desflurane
  3. halothane
  4. enflurane

429. Perioperative blood loss in patient with end-stage renal disease can be decreased by
  1. desmopressin administration
  2. cryoprecipitate
  3. preoperative dialysis (2 to 24 hours preop)
  4. histamine type-2 receptor blocking agents

DIRECTIONS (Questions 430–442): Each of the questions or incomplete statements below is followed by five suggested answers or completions. Select the **one** that is best in each case.

430. Side effects of extracorporeal shock wave lithotripsy (ESWL) include all of the following EXCEPT
    A. hematuria
    B. petechiae
    C. decreased renal function
    D. Goldblatt type of hypertension
    E. lung injury

431. During cystoscopy, the blood pressure in a patient with T_6 paraplegia jumps from 110/60 to 200/110. The heart rate drops from 80 to 46. The increase in blood pressure is most likely due to
    A. parasympathetic vasoconstriction below T_6
    B. sympathetic vasoconstriction above T_6
    C. altered baroreceptor function
    D. sympathetic vasoconstriction below T_6
    E. fluid overload

432. Factors contributing to oliguria during general anesthesia include all of the following EXCEPT
    A. increased concentration of vasopressin
    B. increased concentration of aldosterone
    C. hypotension
    D. hypovolemia
    E. administration of aminoglycoside antibiotics

433. If one were to control autonomic hyperreflexia with antihypertensive agents alone, the best agent would be
    A. sodium nitroprusside
    B. trimethaphan
    C. hydralazine
    D. nifedipine
    E. labetalol

434. Effects of hyponatremia < 115 mEq/L include all of the following EXCEPT
  A. seizures
  B. narrowing of the QRS complex
  C. confusion
  D. depressed myocardial contractility
  E. cardiac dysrhythmias

435. Treatment of the TURP syndrome includes all of the following EXCEPT
  A. mannitol 50 gm IV
  B. furosemide 20 mg IV
  C. supplemental oxygen
  D. hypertonic saline
  E. anticonvulsant

436. An antihypertensive agent that should be avoided in patients with end-stage renal disease is
  A. trimethaphan
  B. sodium nitroprusside
  C. nitroglycerin
  D. propranolol
  E. nifedipine

437. Electrolyte changes that occur secondary to chronic renal failure include all of the following EXCEPT
  A. hyperkalemia
  B. hypercalcemia
  C. hypermagnesemia
  D. metabolic acidosis
  E. hyperphosphatemia

438. The most common postoperative complication in dialysis patients undergoing surgical procedures is
  A. wound infection
  B. hypertension
  C. hyperkalemia
  D. hypotension
  E. shunt thrombosis

439. Visual disturbances after transurethral resection of the prostate are associated with
  A. permanent alterations in vision
  B. normal fundoscopic exam
  C. increased intraocular pressure
  D. normal serum glycine concentrations
  E. sorbitol metabolites

440. The following are contraindications to extracorporeal shock wave lithotripsy EXCEPT
  A. aortic aneurysm
  B. orthopedic hip prosthesis
  C. cardiac pacemaker
  D. morbid obesity
  E. coagulopathy

441. Hypokalemia is a side effect of all of the following diuretics EXCEPT
  A. mannitol
  B. acetazolamide
  C. furosemide
  D. hydrochlorothiazide
  E. spironolactone

442. Appropriate treatment of suspected myoglobinuria includes all of the following EXCEPT
  A. alkalinizing the urine
  B. mannitol IV
  C. hydration
  D. dopamine 3 µg/kg/min IV
  E. acidifying the urine

Anesthesia for Urological Surgery

Answers and Discussion

The authors have made every effort to thoroughly verify the answers to the questions that appear on the preceding pages. As in any text, however, some inaccuracies and ambiguities may occur. If in doubt, please consult the indicated reference. When no page number(s) are cited, the reference is to a journal article or to a refresher course lecture that should be read in its entirety.

The Editors

418. (A) Absorption of the nonionic irrigation fluid is associated with a dilutional hyponatremia and with an increase in intravascular volume. These changes can lead to confusion, headache, coma, and seizures, as well as pulmonary edema. Transient blindness is seen with glycine containing irrigation fluids. (**Ref. 4,** #166)

419. (B) An irrigating solution used for TURP must be a nonionic conducting medium to avoid dispersion of the electrical current. It must also be isosmotic to avoid hemolysis. Cytal (sorbitol 2.7% and mannitol 0.54%) and glycine are the two nonionic and isosmotic irrigating solutions most commonly used. Normal saline conducts electrical current and must be avoided. Sterile water will not conduct a current, but when absorbed will lead to hemolysis and hyponatremia. (**Ref. 36,** p. 2055)

420. (**C**) Atracurium is eliminated by a nonenzymatic degradation that is independent of renal function. Twenty to 30% of a dose of vecuronium is eliminated by the kidneys. Its elimination half-life is prolonged by approximately 50% in anephric patients, converting this short-acting muscle relaxant into a long-acting muscle relaxant. It should be used with caution, however, since there are case reports of prolonged blockade with its use. Pancuronium and gallamine have markedly prolonged elimination half-lives in anephric patients, lasting up to 8.2 and 12.5 hours, respectively. (**Ref. 32,** pp. 1796–1797)

421. (**A**) Renal cell tumors may produce hormones or hormone-like substances that include prostaglandins and parathyroid hormone (causing hypercalcemia), prolactin, renin (causing hypertension), gonadotropins, glucocorticoids (causing Cushing's syndrome), and erythropoietin (erythrocytosis). Thyroid hormone is not produced by renal cell carcinoma. In addition, elevated LFTs and anemia are common in this disease. (**Ref. 22,** pp. 1336–1338)

422. (**A**) Chronic renal failure can decrease thiopental induction requirements by up to 75%. This may be a result of reduced levels of albumin (as in cirrhosis) that will increase the nonbound or nonionized fraction of the drug. Advanced age decreases the thiopental requirement, partly by reducing the volume of distribution. Acidosis, not alkalosis will also increase the nonionized form since the pK of thiopental (7.6) is very close to physiologic pH. (**Ref. 36,** p. 1142; **Ref. 32,** pp. 174–175)

423. (**B**) Prerenal oliguria is associated with physiologic mechanisms that conserve salt and water. Thus, a concentrated urine depleted in sodium is formed. In acute tubular necrosis, the urine osmolality is low (<350 mOsm/L) and the urine Na^+ is high (> 40), reflecting impaired tubular concentrating ability. The fractional excretion of sodium

$$FeNa^+(\%) = \frac{\text{Urine Na} \times \text{Plasma CR}}{\text{Urine CR} \times \text{Plasma Na}} \times 100$$

is thought to be a sensitive marker of prerenal ($FeNa^+$ <1) versus renal ($FeNa^+$ >2) causes of oliguria. (**Ref. 7,** p. 1620)

424. (A) Perioperative bleeding is a common complication of TURP. Foley catheter trauma to raw surfaces of the prostatic bed is one source of bleeding. Another source is dilutional thrombocytopenia caused by absorption of a large volume of irrigating solution. DIC is the most ominous cause of bleeding. Tissue thromboplastin, present in high concentrations in prostatic tissue, may trigger DIC when prostatic particles are released into the bloodstream. In DIC the platelet count and plasma fibrinogen level are low and there is a rise in fibrin degradation products. At autopsy, disseminated microthrombi are found throughout the body. Treatment for DIC is fibrinogen 3 to 4 gm IV followed by heparin 2000 unit bolus and 500 U/hr infusion. FFP and platelets should be given if indicated by the coagulation profile. Platelet function is usually not altered by the absorption of irrigating fluid. (**Ref. 4,** #166)

425. (E) The ECG reflects the toxicity of hyperkalemia more closely than the serum potassium concentration. Tall, peaked T waves, ST segment depression, and widening of the QRS complex are seen. If the potassium concentration increases above 8.0 mEq/L, asystole or other dysrhythmias may occur. Management of hyperkalemia should include the discontinuation of any solutions containing K^+, such as lactated Ringers, penicillin G, and parenteral nutritional fluid. Redistribution of K^+ to the intracellular space can be achieved with an insulin and glucose infusion, or induced alkalosis with $NaHCO_3$ and hyperventilation. Increased excretion of potassium can be achieved with diuretic administration and hydration. Calcium gluconate or calcium chloride given intravenously will acutely antagonize the electrophysiologic effects of K^+. (**Ref. 32,** pp. 1451,1793)

426. (A) Patients without renal disease may excrete up to 150 mg of protein per day, and small amounts may be normal in the urine. Transient proteinuria may be present in several situations, including fever, strenuous exercise, congestive heart failure, seizures, and exposure to extremes of temperature. Massive proteinuria usually implies severe glomerular damage. Glucose is freely filtered at the glomerulus and subsequently is reabsorbed in the proximal tubule. Glycosuria is usually indicative of diabetes mellitus, but may also be the result of rapid IV glucose infusion exceeding the renal threshold. (**Ref. 32,** p. 1792)

427. (E) The causes of perioperative renal failure can be divided into two main groups: (1) those caused by decreased renal perfusion (intravascular volume contraction, cardiopulmonary bypass, aortic cross-clamping, and low cardiac output states), (2) those caused by nephrotoxin exposure (aminoglycosides, radio-contrast agents, anesthetic agents). (**Ref. 36,** p. 306)

428. (D) Enflurane is the only commonly used halogenated inhalational agent that produces a concentration of a significant plasma fluoride ion. Plasma concentrations of 20 to 30 μmol/L can be encountered after enflurane anesthesia. Even though serum concentrations of 50 to 80 μmol/L appear to be necessary to cause the irreversible polyuric renal failure, which is resistant to vasopressin, measurable reductions in the ability of the kidney to concentrate urine have been detected following enflurane anesthesia. Therefore, enflurane should be avoided in patients with renal insufficiency. Desflurane is minimally degraded and has little or no effect on renal blood flow. (**Ref. 36,** p. 307)

429. (E) Abnormal platelet function is the most common clotting abnormality observed in uremic patients. Dialysis partially corrects platelet dysfunction and should be completed within 2 to 24 hours before surgery. Residual heparin from dialysis can result in increased intraoperative bleeding if the dialysis was not completed until two hours prior to surgery. Desmopressin shortens the bleeding time and increases circulating levels of factor VIII/von Willebrand antigen. H_2 blocking agents can help reduce gastrointestinal blood loss caused by stress ulcers, which have a high incidence in dialysis patients. Cryoprecipitate and conjugated estrogens have also been used to decrease the bleeding tendency in uremic patients, although the mechanism of their action is not known. (**Ref. 36,** p. 302)

Answers and Discussion: 427–433 / 251

430. (D) ESWL damages tissues in its path. This can lead to hematuria, petechiae, decreased renal function and injury to lungs, pancreas, and stomach. The Goldblatt type of hypertension due to scarring was once considered a possibility but has not been found to be true. The incidence of new-onset hypertension after ESWL appears to be low, and it is currently uncertain whether there is a link between ESWL and hypertension. (**Ref. 36,** pp. 2057–2059)

431. (D) Autonomic hyperreflexia occurs in 85% of patients with spinal cord lesions above T_5 and can occur in patients with lower spinal cord lesions. Autonomic hyperreflexia is characterized by reflex vasoconstriction due to surgical stimulation below the level of the lesion. Intact baroreceptors cause a reduction in heart rate (vagus) and an inhibition of sympathetic tone above the level of the spinal cord lesion. Thus, a patient with autonomic hyperreflexia will have hypertension, bradycardia, and flushing of the face and neck. (**Ref. 3,** #251)

432. (E) Intraoperative oliguria can result from hemodynamic and/or endocrine factors which lead to an acute reduction in GFR, an acute increase in reabsorption of salt and water, or both. Vasopressin (ADH) is increased during general anesthesia and promotes reabsorption of water in the distal end of the distal convoluted tubule and the collecting ducts. Aldosterone, also increased during general anesthesia, results in the reabsorption of Na^+ in the distal convoluted tubule and collecting ducts. Water passively follows the Na^+ absorption. Alpha agonists and hypotension can reduce GFR and result in decreased urine output. Aminoglycosides cause damage to the renal parenchyma and most often cause a nonoliguric acute renal failure. (**Ref. 7,** p. 1992)

433. (B) Autonomic hyperreflexia is a sudden massive sympathetic discharge with severe hypertension and results from reflex stimulation to the sympathetic neurons in the spinal cord below the level of the lesion. Trimethaphan is a ganglionic blocking agent that has the advantage of blocking reflex vasoconstriction at the ganglionic level, thus inhibiting the reflex. It is used as an intravenous infusion and is titratable. Hydralazine, nifedipine, and labetalol have longer half-lives, which makes their use in this situation difficult. Nitroprusside, the second-best choice, acts directly on vascular smooth muscle. Hypotension between episodes of surgical stimulation may be more prominent with sodium nitroprusside than with a ganglionic blocking agent. (**Ref. 15,** p. 217)

434. **(B)** Hyponatremia can cause disturbances in electrophysiology. ECG changes include widening of the QRS complexes and S-T segment elevation. Myocardial depression and cardiac dysrhythmias also occur. The central nervous system changes include restlessness and confusion. Seizures may appear at serum sodium concentrations near 102 mEq/L. In the TURP syndrome, hypervolemia leading to cerebral edema plays a large role in the CNS symptoms. (**Ref. 7,** p. 116)

435. **(A)** The TURP syndrome is seen near the end of or immediately following transurethral resection of the prostate and is characterized by headache, restlessness, confusion, nausea and vomiting, skeletal muscle twitching, hypertension, and bradycardia. These may progress to hypotension, pulmonary edema (dyspnea and cyanosis), cardiac dysrhythmias, seizures, and death. Hyponatremia and hypervolemia due to intravascular absorption of irrigating solution underlie these features. Treatment is aimed at correcting these underlying physiologic derangements. Supplemental O_2 and positive pressure ventilation (if necessary) will provide supportive therapy for pulmonary edema, while diuresis with a loop diuretic such as furosemide will facilitate removal of extra body water. Mannitol is often used in the irrigating solution. Intravenous mannitol will acutely increase the intravascular volume and may make pulmonary edema worse. If the sodium is <120 mEq/L or the patient shows signs of CNS irritability, hypertonic saline (3% to 5%) at a rate no faster than 100 mL/hr is recommended. Rapid administration of hypertonic saline can be dangerous, leading to pulmonary edema or to a fatal central pontine myelinolysis. If seizures occur, the IV administration of a short-acting anticonvulsant such as midazolam or diazepam is recommended. (**Ref. 4,** #166)

436. **(B)** Sodium nitroprusside, a powerful direct-acting vasodilator, is metabolized via cyanide to thiocyanate. Thiocyanate is cleared slowly by the kidney, and is toxic when levels exceed 10 mg/100 mL. Hypoxia, nausea, tinnitus, muscle spasm, disorientation, and psychosis have been reported at these levels. Trimethaphan, a ganglionic blocking agent, is safe because its action is terminated

enzymatically. Nitroglycerin is rapidly metabolized with less than 1% excreted unchanged in the urine. The calcium channel blocking agents (nifedipine, diltiazem, and verapamil) are metabolized in the liver to inert products. Propranolol is metabolized by the liver, and its activity is not prolonged in a patient with renal failure. Agents with significant renal elimination include methyldopa and guanethidine. The elimination half-life of hydralazine is mildly prolonged in uremic patients. (**Ref. 32,** p. 1798)

436. **(B)** Hypocalcemia (not hypercalcemia) results from the impaired ability of the kidney to synthesize 1,25-dihydroxyvitamin D. Reabsorption of Ca^{++} in the gut is impaired when 1,25-dihydroxyvitamin D is deficient. Hyperphosphatemia facilitates deposition of calcium in the bones and also contributes to hypocalcemia. Tetany is rarely a problem from this cause of hypocalcemia, although it can occur if the patient becomes alkalotic. Calcium gluconate or calcium chloride are usually not required, but if given, they should be administered slowly to prevent intravascular precipitation with phosphates. Hyperkalemia is the most life-threatening electrolyte abnormality. For this reason, dialysis should be done 24 hours prior to surgery and serum K^+ should be less than 5.5 mEq/L prior to induction. Hypermagnesemia occurs from decreased renal elimination and may potentiate nondepolarizing muscle relaxants. Hypermagnesemia that results from chronic renal failure is usually modest and does not cause significant muscle weakness. Excessive ingestion of magnesium, however, can result in significantly elevated serum levels of magnesium. Clinically evident muscle weakness from hypermagnesemia occurs at serum concentations of 4 to 7 mEq/L, and respiratory paralysis occurs at concentrations of 15 mEq/L. Muscular weakness caused by hypermagnesemia can be antagonized with calcium and anticholinesterases. (**Ref. 22,** pp. 2167–2171)

438. **(C)** Hyperkalemia occurs postoperatively in approximately 30% of dialysis patients. Hyperkalemia is the most common indication for dialysis within 24 hours postop. Dialysis within 24 hours prior to the planned procedure is recommended. The other complications—wound infections, hyper- or hypotension, and shunt thrombosis—occur in approximately 10% of the patients. (**Ref. 36,** p. 300)

254 / 16: Anesthesia for Urological Surgery

439. (B) Visual disturbances as a complication of TURP have been reported only when glycine is used in the irrigating fluid and when hyponatremia has occurred. Symptoms include a "dimming of vision" and "light perception only," which can occur up to 6 hours postop and can last up to 12 hours. Fundoscopic exam is normal, and IOP is normal. For this to occur, serum glycine concentrations are usually 30× greater than normal. This condition is fully reversible and no acute management is necessary. Sorbitol is metabolized to glucose and has not been associated with visual disturbances after TURP. (**Ref. 7,** pp. 1161–1163)

440. (D) The contraindications to ESWL include: (1) aortic aneurysm because of calcifications that may absorb energy from the shock wave and lead to rupture or embolizations of plaques; (2) hip prosthesis, because of reflection of the energy waves; (3) coagulopathy, because bleeding is expected from the procedure; and (4) morbid obesity, due to difficulty locating the stone and the gantry supporting the weight. Cardiac pacemakers are generally safe for ESWL, as long as the shock pulses are synchronized with the patient's heartbeat; the patient's heart is monitored during the procedure. Oversensing has occurred in dual-chamber pacemakers. This type of pacemaker may have to be reprogrammed to the single-chamber mode to avoid oversensing. (**Ref. 32,** pp. 1804–1805)

441. (E) Spironolactone is an aldosterone antagonist and its use results in the sparing of K^+. In fact, rare cases of hyperkalemia have been reported with its use. Diuretics that function proximal to the collecting duct can all result in K^+ wasting. Therefore, a K^+ concentration should be checked in all patients taking a diuretic. (**Ref. 15,** p. 908)

442. (E) Myoglobinuria can be caused by a number of conditions. Most important to the anesthesiologist are crush injuries, massive burns, infarctions of muscle, or malignant hyperthermia. Myoglobinuria can lead to acute tubular necrosis associated with the precipitation of myoglobin in the renal tubules. Prevention of ARF in these circumstances encompasses (1) maximizing renal blood flow through judicious hydration and "renal dose" dopamine; (2) promoting diuresis to keep the tubules free of debris; and (3) alkalinization of the urine to prevent formation of myoglobin casts. (**Ref. 22,** pp. 2362–2363)

17
Anesthesia for Ophthalmologic Surgery

DIRECTIONS (Questions 443–460): For each of the questions or incomplete answers below, **one** or **more** of the answers or completions are correct. Select
  A. if only 1, 2, and 3 are correct
  B. if only 1 and 3 are correct
  C. if only 2 and 4 are correct
  D. if only 4 is correct
  E. if all are correct

---

443. The anesthetic objective(s) of managing a patient with penetrating eye injury is (are) to
  1. prevent additional increase in intraocular pressure
  2. avoid an elevation in venous pressure
  3. avoid hypercapnia
  4. avoid a deep level of anesthesia

444. In managing a patient with penetrating eye injury who has recently eaten, choices of the anesthetic plan include
    1. smooth, well-conducted awake intubation
    2. regional anesthesia by performing retrobulbar block
    3. topical anesthesia
    4. rapid sequence induction with cricoid pressure

445. Special concern(s) with strabismus surgery in pediatric patients is (are)
    1. postoperative eye patches
    2. oculocardiac reflex
    3. malignant hyperthermia
    4. postoperative vomiting

446. In a 5-year-old patient with congenital glaucoma, it is safe to use
    1. parenteral atropine as premedication
    2. IV atropine and neostigmine for reversal of muscle relaxants
    3. IV atropine as treatment of oculocardiac reflex
    4. atropine eye drops in preparation for surgery

447. The following condition(s) may have a greater risk of malignant hyperthermia
    1. ptosis
    2. inguinal hernia
    3. strabismus
    4. diaphragmatic hernia

448. Disease(s) that has (have) a strong association with malignant hyperthermia include
    1. Duchenne's muscular dystrophy
    2. familial periodic paralysis
    3. myotonia congenita
    4. myasthenia gravis

449. To produce an acute reduction in intraocular pressure in glaucoma patients, an IV hypertonic solution is used, such as
    1. mannitol
    2. sorbitol
    3. urea
    4. dextran

450. In a patient scheduled for a corneal transplant, general anesthesia is indicated if the patient
  1. is unable to cooperate
  2. is unable to lie flat
  3. has abnormal coagulation profile
  4. has endophthalmitis

451. Acetazolamide (Diamox)
  1. is used to treat open-angle glaucoma
  2. should be avoided in closed-angle glaucoma
  3. should be avoided in hypokalemia
  4. should be avoided in head injury

452. Which of the following statement(s) about the oculocardiac reflex is (are) true?
  1. the reflex is trigemino-vagal
  2. retrobulbar block is not uniformly effective in preventing the reflex
  3. retrobulbar block may precipitate the reflex
  4. the reflex cannot be elicited in an enucleated eye

453. Echothiophate
  1. is a topical long-acting anticholinesterase drug
  2. its systemic absorption leads to inhibition of plasma cholinesterase
  3. is phospholine iodide
  4. is used to maintain mydriasis in the treatment of glaucoma

454. Retrobulbar block complication(s) include
  1. retrobulbar hemorrhage
  2. optic nerve damage
  3. brain stem anesthesia
  4. intraarterial injection

455. Which of the following statements about the effects of anesthetic drugs on intraocular pressure (IOP) is (are) true?
  1. isoflurane lowers IOP
  2. thiopental lowers IOP
  3. fentanyl lowers IOP
  4. etomidate lowers IOP

456. The Valsalva maneuver significantly increases central venous pressure and intraocular pressure. This is due to
1. increased choroidal blood volume
2. distention of orbital vessels
3. interference with aqueous humor drainage
4. increased aqueous humor formation

457. For pediatric strabismus surgery, most anesthesiologists currently favor routine prophylaxis with
1. IV atropine 0.02 mg/kg prior to surgery
2. IM atropine, 0.04 mg/kg 30 minutes prior to surgery
3. IV glycopyrrolate, 0.01 mg/kg prior to surgery
4. oral atropine 0.04 mg/kg one hour prior to surgery

458. If a patient requires re-operation and general anesthesia after intravitreal gas injection
1. N_2O should be avoided for 5 days following air injection
2. N_2O should be avoided for 10 days following sulfur hexafluoride (SF_6) injection
3. N_2O should be avoided for 15 days following octafluorocyclobutane (C_4F_8) injection
4. N_2O should be avoided for 30 days following perfluoropropane (C_3F_8) injection

459. Intraocular pressure is maintained by
1. a dynamic balance between vitreous humor formation and its elimination
2. changes in the choroidal blood volume
3. changes in the vitreous humor volume
4. a dynamic balance between aqueous humor formation and its elimination

460. Increased intraocular pressure secondary to changes in choroidal blood volume occur in response to
1. elevated central venous pressure
2. respiratory acidosis
3. hypoxia
4. metabolic acidosis

DIRECTIONS (Questions 461–470): Each of the questions or incomplete statements below is followed by five suggested answers or completions. Select the **one** that is best in each case.

461. Normal intraocular pressure in humans ranges from
    A. 10 to 25 mm Hg
    B. 15 to 25 mm Hg
    C. 15 to 22 mm Hg
    D. 10 to 22 mm Hg
    E. 10 to 30 mm Hg

462. During general anesthesia for left eye enucleation, the heart rate suddenly drops from 80 to 42 beats per minute. The first action the anesthesiologist should take is to
    A. give IV atropine 0.007 mg/kg body weight
    B. check the end tidal CO_2
    C. check the oxygen saturation
    D. ask the surgeon to stop manipulation
    E. run an ECG strip

463. When intravitreal gas injection is planned during vitrectomy
    A. nitrous oxide should be discontinued 5 min prior to air bubble injection
    B. air should not be used in the inspiratory gas mixture if SF_6 is to be injected in the vitreous
    C. air should not be used in the inspiratory gas mixture if air bubble is to be injected in the vitreous
    D. air should be added to the inspiratory gas mixture once the nitrous oxide is discontinued
    E. nitrous oxide should be discontinued 20 min prior to SF_6 bubble injection

464. Which nerve is not included when performing retrobulbar block?
    A. oculomotor nerve (III)
    B. trochlear nerve (IV)
    C. trigeminal nerve (V)
    D. abducens nerve (VI)
    E. facial nerve (VII)

465. Vitreous humor loss can result from coughing or straining during which type of ocular surgery?
  A. scleral buckle
  B. strabismus surgery
  C. optic nerve sheath decompression
  D. penetrating keratoplasty (PKP)
  E. dacryocystorhinostomy (DCR)

466. What is the most significant factor controlling aqueous humor outflow?
  A. the radius of Fontana's spaces
  B. the viscosity of aqueous humor
  C. the length of Fontana's spaces
  D. the central venous pressure
  E. the intraocular pressure

Questions 467–470: A healthy 10-year-old female is scheduled to undergo strabismus surgery. Immediately following a successful induction and tracheal intubation, the ophthalmologist notices elevated intraocular pressure.

467. Which neuromuscular blocking drug was probably used?
  A. pancuronium
  B. atracurium
  C. succinylcholine
  D. vecuronium
  E. d-tubocurarine

468. For how long will the IOP stay elevated?
  A. 7 min
  B. 17 min
  C. 27 min
  D. 15 min
  E. 3 min

469. For how long should the ophthalmologist wait before performing forced duction test?
  A. 3 min
  B. 5 min

C. 10 min
D. 15 min
E. 20 min

470. What other condition increases intraocular pressure?
A. hypothermia
B. metabolic acidosis
C. respiratory acidosis
D. Fowler position
E. respiratory alkalosis

Anesthesia for Ophthalmologic Surgery

Answers and Discussion

The authors have made every effort to thoroughly verify the answers to the questions that appear on the preceding pages. As in any text, however, some inaccuracies and ambiguities may occur. If in doubt, please consult the indicated reference. When no page number(s) are cited, the reference is to a journal article or to a refresher course lecture that should be read in its entirety.

The Editors

443. (A) Because penetrating eye injuries can result in extrusion of intraocular contents, a major anesthetic objective is to prevent additional increases in intraocular pressure and thus prevent further prolapse and loss of intraocular contents. Other considerations for the patients with an open globe include avoidance of elevated venous pressure from straining or coughing, which can increase intraocular pressure as much as 60 mm Hg. (**Ref. 29,** pp. 186–187)

444. (D) Methods and maneuvers used to protect against aspiration of gastric contents must be assessed relative to their effects on intraocular pressure. Although a well-conducted, extremely smooth awake intubation following topical anesthesia might not increase intraocular pressure, the overwhelming likelihood is that coughing and straining will occur during intubation, resulting in significantly increased intraocular pressure. Performance of retrobulbar block is contraindicated in this setting because extrusion of intraocular contents can result. Topical anesthesia by itself is not sufficient to perform this kind of surgery. (**Ref. 29,** p.186)

445. (E) There are many concerns when caring for young patients undergoing strabismus surgery. The child should understand that one or both eyes may be patched after surgery. Occluded or diminished vision secondary to patches or ointment may terrify the child as he or she emerges from anesthesia. There is also a high incidence of oculocardiac reflex-induced dysrhythmias, an increased incidence of malignant hyperthermia, and postoperative nausea and vomiting. (**Ref. 29,** p.191)

446. (A) Atropine premedication in the doses used clinically has no effect on intraocular pressure in either open- or closed-angle glaucoma. IV atropine and neostigmine may be safely used to reverse muscular blockade in patients with glaucoma. Topical atropine should be avoided in all patients with glaucoma. (**Ref. 29,** p.199)

447. (A) Even mild and common muscle problems may increase the risk of malignant hyperthermia. These conditions include inguinal hernia, ptosis, strabismus, generalized muscle bulk loss, localized muscle weakness, and even a history of muscle cramps, especially if linked with caffeine ingestion. (**Ref. 29,** p.194)

448. (B) Diseases that have a strong association with malignant hyperthermia (MH) include Duchenne's muscular dystrophy and Becker's muscular dystrophy, as well as central core disease, myotonia congenita, and arthrogryposis. There is some debate whether osteogenesis imperfecta has a strong link with MH. Most anesthesiologists avoid drugs that might trigger MH in all of the aforementioned conditions. (**Ref. 29,** p. 194)

449. (E) IV hypertonic solutions, such as dextran, urea, mannitol, and sorbitol, elevate plasma osmotic pressure relative to aqueous humor pressure and produce an acute, albeit temporary, reduction in intraocular pressure, as shown by the following equation:

$$IOP = K[(Opaq - Opal) + CP]$$

K = coefficient of outflow, Opaq = osmotic pressure of aqueous humor, Opal = osmotic pressure of plasma, CP = capillary pressure. **(Ref. 29, p. 231)**

450. (A) Relative contraindications to local anesthesia include ruptured globe, infection at or near the site of injection, abnormal coagulation or bleeding profile, inability to communicate (language barrier or deafness), inability to lie flat, inability to cooperate (e.g., excessive anxiety, claustrophobia), chronic coughing or tremor and patient refusal. Endophthalmitis is an infection within the eyeball; local anesthesia is not contraindicated. **(Ref. 29, p. 273)**

451. (B) Acetazolamide (Diamox), is a sulfonamide derivative. It inhibits carbonic anhydrase, thus depressing the sodium pump mechanism responsible for secretion of aqueous humor. It is taken orally to treat open-angle glaucoma. Because renal carbonic anhydrase activity is also affected, bicarbonate diuresis with concomitant losses of water, sodium, and potassium occurs with chronic therapy. **(Ref. 29, pp. 232, 263)**

452. (A) The oculocardiac reflex is trigemino-vagal. The afferent limb is from orbital contents to the ciliary ganglion to the ophthalmic division of the trigeminal nerve to the sensory nucleus of the trigeminal nerve near the fourth ventricle. The efferent limb is via the vagus nerve. Retrobulbar block is not uniformly effective in preventing the reflex. In fact, retrobulbar block may precipitate the response. The reflex may be elicited by direct pressure on the tissues remaining in the orbital apex after enucleation. **(Ref. 36, p. 2243; Ref. 7, p. 1100)**

453. (A) Echothiophate or phospholine iodide is a topical long-acting anticholinesterase drug used to maintain miosis in the treatment of glaucoma. Systemic absorption leads to inhibition of plasma cholinesterase. Subsequent administration of succinylcholine causes prolonged muscle paralysis. Return to normal enzyme activity may take 4 to 6 weeks after discontinuation of the drug. (**Ref. 36,** p. 2244)

454. **(E)** The most common complication of retrobulbar block is retrobulbar hemorrhage. Proptosis and subconjunctival ecchymosis will be seen. Accidental intra-arterial injection can give high brain levels via retrograde flow in the internal carotid. This can result in CNS excitation and convulsions. Obtundation and respiratory arrest have been reported and are thought to be caused by injection into the optic nerve sheath, which is continuous with the subarachnoid space. (**Ref. 36,** p. 2247)

455. **(E)** Inhalation anesthetics cause dose-related decreases in IOP. Virtually all CNS depressants, including barbiturates, neuroleptics, opioids, tranquilizers, and hypnotics lower IOP in both normal and glaucomatous eyes. Etomidate, despite its proclivity to produce pain on intravenous injection and skeletal muscle movement, is associated with a significant reduction in IOP. (**Ref. 7,** p. 1099)

456. **(A)** If venous return from the eye is disturbed at any point from Schlemm's canal to the right atrium, intraocular pressure increases substantially. This is due to both increased intraocular blood volume and to the distention of the orbital vessels, as well as to interference with aqueous humor drainage. Straining, vomiting, and coughing increase venous pressure and can raise intraocular pressure as much as 40 mm Hg or more. (**Ref. 7,** p. 1098)

457. **(B)** In an effort to reduce the incidence of oculocardiac reflex, the current popular practice favors administration of IV atropine, 0.02 mg/kg, before commencing surgery. Alternatively, glycopyrrolate, 0.01 mg/kg, administered IV, may be associated with less tachycardia than atropine does. The oral route is not popular because of its slower absorption and erratic efficacy. (**Ref. 7,** p. 1101)

458. (E) If a patient requires reoperation and general anesthesia after intravitreal gas injection, N_2O should be avoided for 5 days following air injection, for 10 days following sulfurhexafluoride (SF_6) injection. Octafluorocyclobutane (C_4F_8) remains in the vitreous cavity for more than 13 days, and perfluoropropane (C_3F_8) lingers for longer than 30 days. (**Ref. 7,** p. 1103)

459. (C) The main physiologic determinant of intraocular pressure is the dynamic balance between the production of aqueous humor in the ciliary body and its eventual elimination into the episcleral venous system via the spaces of Fontana and the canal of Schlemm. Changes in choroidal blood volume also affect the intraocular pressure significantly. (**Ref. 32,** p. 2004)

460. (A) If venous return from the eye is disturbed at any point from Schlemm's canal to the right atrium, intraocular pressure (IOP) will increase substantially. This is caused by both intraocular blood volume and distention of the ocular vessels, as well as by interference with aqueous drainage. Coughing, bucking, vomiting and the Valsalva maneuver greatly increase venous pressure and thus increase intraocular pressure. Intraocular vascular tone is predominantly affected by carbon dioxide and by control areas in the diencephalon. The increased intraocular pressure associated with hypoventilation and hypercarbia (respiratory acidosis) occurs as the result of vasodilation of the choroidal blood vessels and increases in central venous pressure. A linear relationship exists between IOP and $PaCO_2$. Choroidal circulation is also sensitive to changes in $PaCO_2$. Hypoxia induces choroidal vasodilation and thus also increases intraocular pressure. Metabolic acidosis reduces choroidal blood volume and intraocular pressure. Metabolic alkalosis increases them. (**Ref. 29,** p. 185; **Ref. 32,** p. 2004)

461. (D) Normal intraocular pressure in humans ranges from 10 to 22 mm Hg. This level fluctuates 1 to 2 mm Hg with each cardiac contraction and 2 to 5 mm Hg with diurnal variation. (**Ref. 29,** p. 183)

462. (D) Recommended treatment for a single episode of oculocardiac reflex is as follows:

Request the surgeon to stop manipulation
Assess ventilatory status
If severe or persistent bradycardia is present, administer intravenous atropine in 0.007 mg/kg increments
(Ref. 36, p. 2243)

463. (E) Ophthalmologists sometimes inject a small bubble of gas into the vitreal cavity during surgical reattachment of the retina. The gases commonly used, SF_6 and C_3F_8, are inert, very insoluble in water, and poorly diffusible. N_2O is 117 times more diffusible than SF_6 and rapidly enters the gas bubble. Because washout of N_2O from the lung is 90% complete within 10 minutes, administration of N_2O should be discontinued at least 20 minutes before an intravitreal injection of gas. **(Ref. 32, pp. 2005–2006)**

464. (E) The superior orbital fissure transmits the superior and inferior branches of the oculomotor nerve; the lacrimal, frontal, and nasociliary branches of the trigeminal nerve; and the trochlear and abducens nerves. All these nerves will be blocked when performing a retrobulbar block. This is accomplished by injecting a local anesthetic solution behind the bulb into the muscle cone formed by the extraocular muscles. The facial nerve has to be blocked separately, since it does not run through the orbit. **(Ref. 29, pp. 176, 235)**

465. (D) If coughing or straining occurs during ocular surgery when the eye is open, as in cataract extraction or in penetrating keratoplasty (corneal transplant), the result may be a disastrous expulsive hemorrhage or loss of vitreous, secondary to suddenly increased intraocular pressure. Scleral buckling, strabismus surgery, optic nerve sheath decompression, and DCR are all extraocular surgical procedures (i.e., the eye is not open, and so there is no danger of expulsion of ocular contents, should the IOP rise suddenly). **(Ref. 7, p. 1098)**

466. (A) The most significant factor controlling aqueous humor outflow is the diameter of Fontana's spaces as illustrated by the following equation:

$$A = r^4 \times (P_{iop} - P_v)/8\mu L,$$

where

A = volume of aqueous outflow per unit of time
r = radius of Fontana's spaces
P_{iop} = intraocular pressure
P_v = venous pressure
μ = viscosity
L = length of Fontana's spaces

(**Ref. 7,** p. 1098)

467. (C) The nondepolarizing neuromuscular blocking agents are associated with a decrease or with no change in the IOP. Curare and pancuronium have been reported to lower IOP, whereas both atracurium and vecuronium are believed to have no intrinsic effect on IOP. The ocular muscles differ anatomically from the skeletal muscles in having a population of muscle fibers with multiple motor-nerve endings. Whereas skeletal muscles respond to depolarizing drugs with flaccid paralysis, the ocular response to succinylcholine is one of sustained tonic contracture. A variety of maneuvers, including prior treatment with a nondepolarizing neuromuscular blocking agent, self-taming with succinylcholine, acetazolamide, propranolol, lidocaine, and diazepam have been advocated to prevent the increase in IOP produced by succinylcholine. Although some attenuation of the pressure increase may ensue, none of these drugs consistently prevents the ocular hypertensive response. (**Ref. 7,** p. 1100)

468. (A) IV succinylcholine induces an intraocular pressure increase of about 8 mm Hg within 1 to 4 minutes. Within 7 minutes, intraocular pressure returns to baseline. (**Ref. 7,** p. 1100)

469. (E) It is suggested to wait 20 min after administration of succinylcholine before performing the forced duction test. (**Ref. 7,** p. 1100)

470. (C) Respiratory acidosis increases both choroidal blood volume and intraocular pressure, whereas respiratory alkalosis does the opposite. Metabolic acidosis reduces choroidal blood volume and intraocular pressure, and metabolic alkalosis increases them. Hypothermia lowers intraocular pressure by decreasing aqueous humor formation and by vasoconstriction. Fowler position (head up) decreases intraocular pressure. (**Ref. 29,** p. 185)

18

Anesthesia for Transplant Surgery

DIRECTIONS (Questions 471–480): Each of the questions or incomplete statements below is followed by five suggested answers or completions. Select the **one** that is best in each case.

471. The proper order of organ ischemia time for transplantation is (shortest to longest)
   A. heart, kidney, liver
   B. liver, heart, kidney
   C. kidney, liver, heart
   D. heart, liver, kidney
   E. lung, liver, brain

472. Which of the following drugs is best for rapid sequence intubation in a patient with renal failure?
   A. high-dose vecuronium
   B. high-dose atracurium
   C. priming dose vecuronium
   D. rocuronium
   E. succinylcholine

473. Organs are harvested in which of the following orders?
   A. liver, heart, kidney
   B. liver, kidney, heart
   C. heart, kidney, liver
   D. heart, liver, kidney
   E. kidney, heart, liver

474. CMV positive organs may be transplanted
   A. never
   B. always
   C. into CMV negative recipients
   D. into CMV positive recipients
   E. into hepatitis B positive recipients

475. The most common cause of death in patients with CRF is
   A. anesthesia related
   B. sepsis
   C. uremia
   D. anemia
   E. coronary artery disease

476. Portal hypertension during the anhepatic phase of liver transplantation can be decreased by
   A. induced hypotension
   B. surgical bleeding
   C. veno-venous bypass
   D. nasogastric suction
   E. hypoventilation

477. In a transplanted heart, which of the following drugs is least effective in increasing the heart rate?
   A. isoproterenol
   B. epinephrine
   C. dobutamine
   D. dopamine
   E. atropine

478. Which of the following therapies remove excess potassium from a patient in renal failure?
   A. IV calcium chloride
   B. hemodialysis
   C. hyperventilation
   D. IV insulin
   E. IV insulin and glucose

479. Which of the following is NOT true for lung transplantation?
   A. right side is preferred for single lung transplantation
   B. the lung is the only transplanted organ exposed to the external environment
   C. PEEP, CPAP, and pulmonary artery ligation may improve oxygenation
   D. cardiopulmonary bypass may be necessary in pulmonary hypertension
   E. CPB is necessary in "en bloc" double lung transplant

480. In a denervated, post-transplanted heart, which of the following drugs will change the heart rate?
   A. atropine
   B. neostigmine
   C. pancuronium
   D. ephedrine
   E. edrophonium

DIRECTIONS (Questions 481–498): For each of the questions or incomplete answers below, **one** or **more** of the answers or completions are correct. Select
- **A.** if only 1, 2, and 3 are correct
- **B.** if only 1 and 3 are correct
- **C.** if only 2 and 4 are correct
- **D.** if only 4 is correct
- **E.** if all are correct

481. Which of the following therapies is likely to be ineffective in a bradycardic arrest of an ASA VI organ donor?
    1. isoproterenol
    2. epinephrine
    3. pacing
    4. atropine

482. Organ preservation is prolonged by which of the following measures?
    1. using high-potassium solutions to decrease cellular respiration
    2. using free-radical scavengers to prevent damage
    3. using hypothermia to decrease cellular respiration
    4. using high-calcium solutions to maintain organ function

483. Which of the following is (are) contraindication(s) to organ transplantation?
    1. diabetes
    2. incurable malignancy
    3. history of alcohol abuse
    4. active infection

484. Massive blood replacement during liver transplantation is complicated by
    1. hypothermia
    2. dilution of coagulation factors
    3. hypocalcemia
    4. myocardial depression

274 / 18: Anesthesia for Transplant Surgery

485. Signs of renal rejection include
1. hyperthermia
2. disseminated intravascular coagulation
3. decreased urine output
4. hypoglycemia

486. Appropriate anesthetic management for donor nephrectomy could include
1. neuromuscular blocking drugs
2. volatile anesthetics
3. potent narcotics
4. fluid restriction

487. Treatment of hypertension in the prerenal transplant patient includes
1. calcium channel blockers
2. beta blockers
3. prazosin
4. nephrectomy

488. Which of the following is (are) true for renal transplantation?
1. patients are at increased risk for infection
2. surgery should be delayed until after dialysis
3. patients are sick
4. the aorta is cross-clamped to allow for anastomosis of the renal artery

489. Liver transplant can cure which of the following diseases?
1. hemophilia A
2. Wilson's disease
3. alpha$_1$–antitrypsin deficiency
4. sickle cell disease

490. Which of the following prevents the definitive diagnosis of brain death?
1. hyponatremia
2. barbiturates
3. seizures
4. deep hypothermia

491. Which of the following drugs have potentially toxic metabolites?
   1. meperidine
   2. atracurium
   3. enflurane
   4. gallamine

492. Peritoneal dialysis uses which of the following?
   1. hypertonic solutions
   2. hypotonic solutions
   3. peritoneal membrane
   4. intravascular cannulas

493. Liver synthetic function is tested by which of the following?
   1. AST
   2. prothrombin time
   3. ALT
   4. serum albumin

494. Severe liver disease is often associated with
   1. hyponatremia
   2. hypernatremia
   3. hypokalemia
   4. normal water balance

495. Contraindications to lung transplant include
   1. neuromuscular disease
   2. advanced right ventricular failure
   3. glucocorticoid dependence
   4. increased oxygen requirements

496. Which of the following is (are) contraindication(s) to heart transplant?
   1. active infection
   2. viral cardiomyopathy
   3. severe pulmonary hypertension
   4. NYHA Class IV

497. Postoperative considerations in the patient with a transplanted lung include
1. infection
2. airway anastomosis
3. disruption of pulmonary lymphatic drainage
4. denervation of the implanted lung

498. Cyclosporine
1. is nephrotoxic
2. can induce hypertension in heart transplant patients
3. may cause seizures
4. is contraindicated in renal transplant recipients

Anesthesia for Transplant Surgery

Answers and Discussion

The authors have made every effort to thoroughly verify the answers to the questions that appear on the preceding pages. As in any text, however, some inaccuracies and ambiguities may occur. If in doubt, please consult the indicated reference. When no page number(s) are cited, the reference is to a journal article or to a refresher course lecture that should be read in its entirety.

The Editors

471. (D) The maximum permissible ischemia time for hearts is 4 to 6 hours, for livers up to 24 hours, and for kidneys up to 48 hours. Organ death occurs, since the ex vivo organ is without oxygen and nutrients. This leads to anaerobic metabolism, accumulation of acids and metabolites, eventual failure of membrane ion pumps, and cell death associated with influx of calcium. Reperfusion further insults the organ with the formation of free radicals. Preservation strategies include decreasing the metabolic rate with cold, high K^+ solutions and decreasing free radical formation by including free radical scavengers and synthesis blockers. (**Ref. 7,** pp. 1481–1482)

472. (E) Succinylcholine, although it may increase the serum potassium, this increase is not greater in patients with renal failure than in any other patient (0.5 mEq/L). Serum cholinesterase levels are adequate to break down the succinylcholine and the duration of action is not prolonged. (**Ref. 7,** pp. 1141, 1487)

473. (D) Harvesting should be done in the order of their maximum permissible ischemia times. This is done in order to minimize the amount of damage the organ will receive during the ischemic periods (see answer 471 above). (**Ref. 7,** pp. 1481–1482)

474. (D) When the CMV status of the recipient is the same as that of the donor, the recipient should have the antibodies necessary to prevent reinfection. This helps to increase the available pool of organ donors, which is currently the limiting factor in organ transplantation. (**Ref. 7,** p. 1479)

475. (B) Sepsis. The anemia is generally well tolerated, the uremia can be satisfactorily treated with dialysis, the anesthetic mortality is low, and the coronary artery disease is a progressive and usually not acute problem. Sepsis, however, leading to multiorgan failure is deadly. Therefore, as anesthesiologists, we should be quite concerned about the possibility of sepsis and make sure that all indwelling catheters are placed with the most rigid aseptic technique in renal failure patients. (**Ref. 40,** pp. 421–427)

476. (C) Veno-venous bypass . Portal hypertension can cause back pressure on the organs in the portal system, leading to decreased perfusion and to an increase in the release of toxic metabolites and free radicals. Induced hypotension may decrease the portal pressures to normal, but the gradient for perfusion would also be decreased. (**Ref. 36,** pp. 2025–2027)

477. (E) Atropine will be the least effective of these drugs, since the heart is denervated. In the immediate postoperative period most transplanted hearts are paced. Any direct acting beta-adrenergic agonist should increase the heart rate by directly stimulating the heart. (**Ref. 7,** pp. 1504–1506)

478. (B) Hemodialysis. Hyperventilation, IV insulin, and glucose redistribute extracellular potassium into the intracellular space. This may be important in the acute treatment of dysrhythmias, but the total body stores of potassium remain high and can redistribute to cause problems. IV calcium provides a short-term antagonism of the electrophysiologic effects of high plasma concentrations of potassium, but it also does not remove the excess potassium. (**Ref. 40,** p. 458)

479. **(A)** The left side is preferred because of surgical considerations: the left pulmonary veins are more accessible, the left bronchus is longer, and the left chest can better accommodate an oversize lung. Lung transplants are unique in that the transplanted organ must be in contact with the external environment in addition to the patient's internal milieu. By mechanically decreasing shunt, PEEP, CPAP, and pulmonary artery ligation may improve oxygenation. Cardiopulmonary bypass may be necessary as a result of technical considerations or to heart failure. (**Ref. 7,** pp. 1496–1499)

480. **(D)** Ephedrine. All the others act indirectly through the vagus. Atropine is a muscarinic blocker, pancuronium has weak vagolytic properties, and neostigmine and edrophonium increase acetylcholine levels by blocking pseudocholinesterase. The ephedrine response may be diminished, but the heart rate should increase. (**Ref. 7,** pp. 1504–1506)

481. **(D)** Atropine will be ineffective. Theoretically, loss of the vagal nucleus in the CNS abolishes the vagal tone of the heart and minimizes the effects of vagolytic drugs. The other drugs (isoproterenol, epinephrine) and pacing act directly on the myocardium. (**Ref. 7,** 1504–1506)

482. **(A)** High levels of potassium and hypothermia both decrease cellular respiration and prolong ischemia time. Mannitol and other drugs may scavenge toxic free radicals. High calcium levels may lead to cellular death. Different combinations of electrolytes and drugs are used for different organ preservation solutions. (**Ref. 7,** pp. 1481–1482)

483. **(C)** Renal transplants have been successful in diabetic patients. Although this is a controversial issue, a history of previous alcoholism is not viewed as a medical contraindication. Active infection precludes the use of immunosuppressive drugs, which are required for successful transplantation. Incurable tumors generally preclude transplantation since the patient would not live long enough to benefit from the transplant. (Ref. 7, pp. 1486–1493)

484. **(E)** Hypothermia can occur because of the massive fluid replacement, which then also dilutes the coagulation factors. The citrate anticoagulant in blood products binds calcium, causing hypocalcemia. This may become a problem in the patient with a poorly functional or nonfunctional liver since this liver cannot rapidly metabolize the citrate. Hypocalcemia can secondarily affect myocardial function. (Ref. 40, p. 378)

485. **(A)** Renal rejection results in hyperthermia and DIC by activating the immune system, which then in turn destroys kidney function. This results in decreased urine output. The kidney, although it has glycogen stores, is not a significant source of glucose. (Ref. 40, p. 440)

486. **(A)** The choice of anesthesia does not appear to be critical to the outcome of the transplant. Maintaining hydration is important, since renal function depends to some extent upon preload. A large variety of anesthetic techniques and drugs have been used successfully. (Ref. 32, pp. 1800–1802)

487. **(E)** Hypertension is a common problem in renal failure. It is related to the loss of the renal mechanisms for the control of blood pressure and volume status. Initial treatment involves pharmacotherapy of the hypertension, but when hypertension is severe and refractory to treatment, nephrectomy becomes an option. Nephrectomy decreases blood pressure by decreasing the activity of the renin-angiotensin system. (Ref. 32, pp. 1798–1801)

488. **(A)** Because the preoperative uremic state and the postoperative immunosuppression, renal transplant patients are more susceptible to infection. Since the cold ischemia time for kidneys is over 24 hours, the surgery is urgent rather than emergent, and the patient's condition should be optimized prior to surgery. This includes taking the time to dialyze the patient, if appropriate. The anastomosis is done well below the native renal arteries and should not require cross-clamping. (Ref. 32, pp. 1798–1802)

489. (A) Those diseases caused by a genetic defect in liver protein synthesis will be cured by liver transplant. Therefore, the proteins that are involved in hemophilia A, Wilson's disease, and alpha$_1$-antitrypsin deficiency will be restored. Sickle cell disease is due to an abnormal hemoglobin molecule that is produced by bone marrow cells. (**Ref. 22,** pp. 1501–1504)

490. (C) Barbiturates and deep hypothermia can depress EEG and cerebral function in a reversible manner. This is the basis for the statement that the patients are not dead until they're warm and dead. Brain death is an irreversible process. (**Ref. 7,** pp. 1626–1627)

491. (A) Meperidine is metabolized to normeperidine (renally excreted), which can cause seizures. Atracurium eventually degrades to laudanosine, which is potentially neurotoxic. Enflurane is defluorinated, resulting in fluoride ions that can be nephrotoxic (not clinically seen but theoretically possible). Methoxyflurane (no longer in use) has been associated with a high-output renal failure. (**Ref. 41,** pp. 57, 84, 205–206)

492. (A) Peritoneal dialysis can use either hyper- or hypotonic solutions, depending on the volume status of the patient. The peritoneal membrane serves as the dialysis membrane for exchange. Hypertonic solutions draw fluid out of the patient, whereas hypotonic solutions adds volume. No IV is needed. (**Ref. 32,** pp. 1800–1801)

493. (C) Prothrombin time and albumin are tests for the synthetic functions of the liver. AST and ALT increase with injury. This difference is important since patients with end-stage liver disease may have normal circulating enzyme levels but have little remaining synthetic liver function. Patients with acute liver injury may have good functional reserves but very high levels of circulating AST and ALT. (**Ref. 36,** pp. 317–320)

494. (A) Both hypo- and hypernatremia are seen, as well as hypokalemia. Water balance derangements play a part as well as electrolyte derangements. Excess loss of water can contribute to hypernatremia. Renal failure is seen in 50% to 75% of patients dying of cirrhosis. (**Ref. 36,** pp. 2008–2009)

495. **(A)** Patients with neuromuscular disease will have a poor recovery. Patients with RV failure will not tolerate surgery well, and patients receiving glucocorticoids will have impaired healing. Increasing oxygen requirements are an indication for transplantation. (**Ref. 7,** pp. 1496–1499)

496. **(B)** Active infection prevents immunosuppression and leads to rejection. Severe pulmonary hypertension causes acute right heart failure in the new heart. Both viral cardiomyopathy and severe dysfunction from other causes are indications for transplant. (**Ref. 7,** pp. 1492–1496)

497. **(E)** Infection is the most common problem in transplant patients due to the high degree of immunosuppression. Airway anastomoses are important in the immediate postoperative period. Disruption of pulmonary lymphatic drainage can result in reimplantation pulmonary edema and decreased lung function. Denervation of the implanted lung is a consideration, since this would result in diminished airway reflexes (little evidence exists for its clinical importance). (**Ref. 36,** pp. 1867–1875)

498. **(A)** Cyclosporine is nephrotoxic, but it is still used for immunosuppression in renal transplant patients because of its great efficacy in preventing rejection. Hypertension and seizures are other known side effects. (**Ref. 41,** pp. 425–426)

19

Anesthesia for Obstetrics

DIRECTIONS (Questions 499–517): Each of the questions or incomplete statements below is followed by five suggested answers or completions. Select the **one** that is best in each case.

---

499. Fetal presentation is
   A. the distance between the presenting fetal part to an imaginary line drawn between the maternal ischial spines
   B. the relationship of the fetal head to the long axis of the fetus
   C. the relationship of the long axis of the fetus to the long axis of the mother
   D. the relationship of fetal skull suture lines to the maternal pelvic inlet
   E. the relationship of the fetal skull suture lines to the long axis of the mother

500. All of the following are types of breech presentation EXCEPT
   A. complete breech
   B. transverse breech
   C. frank breech
   D. incomplete breech
   E. footling breech

501. Umbilical cord prolapse is most common in
   A. cephalic presentation
   B. complete breech
   C. footling breech
   D. frank breech
   E. transverse presentation

502. In the vaginal delivery of a breech presentation
   A. supplemental maternal oxygen should be avoided for fear of harming the fetus
   B. narcotics should be avoided at all stages of labor
   C. a saddle block should be administered early in labor
   D. relaxation of the perineum is important
   E. an assisted instrumental delivery is remote

503. The pain of labor in the first stage is primarily mediated via the following spinal nerve roots
   A. $T_{10}, T_{11}, T_{12}, L_1$
   B. T_7, T_8, T_9
   C. S_2, S_3, S_4
   D. T_4, T_5, T_6
   E. T_{11}, T_{12}, L_1, L_2

504. The pain of labor in the second stage is mediated primarily via which of the following spinal nerve roots
   A. L_4, L_5, S_1
   B. S_2, S_3, S_4
   C. L_5, S_1, S_2
   D. $T_{10}, T_{11}, T_{12}, L_1$
   E. L_3, L_4, L_5

505. Regional techniques that can be used to alleviate pain during the first stage of labor include all of the following EXCEPT
   A. bilateral pudendal nerve block
   B. bilateral paracervical block
   C. epidural block
   D. subarachnoid block
   E. lumbar sympathetic block

506. A bilateral paracervical nerve block will provide analgesia to
    A. the anus
    B. the perineum
    C. the labium majora
    D. the cervix and lower uterine segment
    E. the vaginal wall

507. An epidural needle reaches the epidural space in the midline by traversing ligaments in the following order
    A. supraspinous, interspinous, ligamentum flavum
    B. interspinous, supraspinous, ligamentum flavum
    C. supraspinous, ligamentum flavum, interspinous
    D. interspinous, ligamentum flavum, supraspinous
    E. ligamentum flavum, supraspinous, interspinous

508. All of the following are true about the use of epidural opioids for labor analgesia EXCEPT
    A. epidural opioids are most effective in alleviating visceral pain
    B. epidural opioids are very effective in alleviating somatic pain
    C. rapidly acting epidural opioids have greater lipid solubility
    D. epidural opioids partly modulate pain transmission at the level of the substantia gelatinosa in the dorsal horn of the spinal cord
    E. the more hydrophilic epidural opioids have a longer duration of action

509. The most appropriate local anesthetic to use for epidural anesthesia for cesarean section for fetal distress is
    A. lidocaine
    B. bupivacaine
    C. 2-chloroprocaine
    D. mepivacaine
    E. procaine

510. The period of organogenesis in the developing human fetus and the most vulnerable period with respect to exposure of the fetus to anesthetic agents is
    A. day 7 through 15
    B. day 15 through 50
    C. day 90 through 280
    D. day 1 through 7
    E. day 1 through 50

511. Patients most predisposed to placenta accreta and requiring emergency hysterectomy to control hemorrhage at the time of cesarean delivery are
    A. patients with a history of placenta previa
    B. patients with a history of previous low transverse cesarean sections
    C. patients with a placenta previa and a history of a previous low transverse cesarean section
    D. patients with a complete placenta previa
    E. patients with a complete abruptio placentae

512. Anesthetic-related maternal mortality in the United States is now most often due to
    A. hemorrhage
    B. airway problems
    C. total spinals
    D. seizures from local anesthetic toxicity
    E. drug error

513. The usual blood loss with a normal vaginal or cesarean delivery respectively is
    A. 600–800 mL, 1200–1400 mL
    B. 300–400 mL, 700–800 mL
    C. 200–300 mL, 600–700 mL
    D. 400–600 mL, 800–1200 mL
    E. 100–200 mL, 400–500 mL

514. The chief side effects of intraspinal narcotics include all of the following EXCEPT
    A. pruritus
    B. constipation

C. nausea and vomiting
D. late respiratory depression
E. urinary retention

515. A 25-year-old gravida 1, para 0, at 32 weeks' gestation is admitted with painful vaginal bleeding. She reports the use of cocaine prior to the onset of the vaginal bleeding. Her blood pressure is 160/110, pulse of 120, repetitive uterine contractions with elevated basal tone, and late decelerations are noted on the fetal heart rate tracing. The most likely diagnosis is
    A. uterine rupture
    B. abruptio placenta
    C. placenta previa
    D. preeclampsia
    E. vaso previa

516. Oxygenated blood returns from the placenta and is delivered to the fetal heart and brain via the
    A. umbilical artery, hepatic vein, left atrium via foramen ovale, and left ventricle
    B. umbilical vein, hepatic vein, left atrium via foramen ovale, left ventricle
    C. umbilical vein, ductus venosus, left atrium via foramen ovale, left ventricle
    D. umbilical artery, ductus venosus, left atrium via foramen ovale, left ventricle
    E. umbilical vein, hepatic artery, left atrium via foramen ovale, left ventricle

517. Neonatal outcome following delivery by cesarean section under regional anesthesia is most directly related to
    A. uterine incision to delivery time
    B. anesthetic induction to delivery time
    C. transient hypotension treated promptly
    D. maternal administration of supplemental oxygen during delivery
    E. skin incision to delivery time

288 / 19: Anesthesia for Obstetrics

DIRECTIONS (Questions 518–529): For each of the questions or incomplete answers below, **one** or **more** of the answers or completions are correct. Select
- **A.** if only 1, 2, and 3 are correct
- **B.** if only 1 and 3 are correct
- **C.** if only 2 and 4 are correct
- **D.** if only 4 is correct
- **E.** if all are correct

518. The definition of preeclampsia includes
   1. hypertension
   2. proteinuria
   3. edema
   4. seizures

519. Which of the following laboratory results would be consistent with a diagnosis of preeclampsia?
   1. hematocrit of 40%
   2. serum glucose less than 50
   3. platelet count less than 100,000
   4. serum sodium of 150 mEq per liter

520. The following should be anticipated by the anesthesiologist when administering a general anesthetic to the severe preeclamptic patient receiving magnesium sulfate
   1. increased upper airway edema
   2. prolonged action of following succinylcholine
   3. marked hypertension with intubation, surgical stimulation, and emergence from general anesthesia
   4. increased MAC compared to normal pregnant patients

521. Which of the following characterize the hemodynamic changes associated with preeclampsia?
   1. decreased systemic vascular resistance
   2. decreased intravascular volume
   3. increased intravascular volume
   4. increased systemic vascular resistance

522. All of the following are true in the preeclamptic patient, EXCEPT
1. the incidence of abruptio placenta is increased
2. the uterus is hyperactive and sensitive to oxytocin
3. uterine and placental blood flow are decreased by 50% to 70%
4. the leading cause of maternal death in preeclampsia is cardiac failure

523. Elevated serum magnesium levels are associated with
1. generalized muscle weakness
2. respiratory depression
3. cardiac depression
4. decreased plasma cholinesterase activity

524. A 22-year-old gravida 1, para 0, term, healthy parturient is scheduled for an emergency cesarean section for fetal distress. It is important that adequate denitrogenation occur prior to induction because
1. a pregnant patient's PO_2 desaturates more rapidly than does a nonpregnant patient's following apnea
2. functional residual capacity is decreased
3. oxygen consumption is increased
4. minute alveolar ventilation is decreased

525. A pregnant patient at term complains of dizziness, nausea, and sweating when lying flat on her back. These symptoms are probably secondary to
1. decreased maternal cardiac preload
2. hypoglycemia
3. inferior vena cava obstruction
4. hypocarbia

526. The cardiovascular changes associated with pregnancy include
1. increased total blood volume
2. increased cardiac output
3. decreased total peripheral resistance
4. normal central venous pressure

527. The parturient at term is considered to be at risk for pulmonary aspiration. The following measures can be taken to prevent aspiration pneumonitis in the pregnant patient EXCEPT
   1. cricoid pressure
   2. administration of an H_2 blocker and/or metoclopramide if time permits
   3. rapid sequence induction and intubation
   4. administration of a particulate antacid

528. Increasing the pH of local anesthetic solution results in
   1. a greater portion of the molecule existing in the ionized form
   2. a greater portion of the molecule existing in the unionized form
   3. onset time is increased
   4. onset time is decreased

529. All of the following act to decrease the incidence of the development of a postdural puncture headache in women of childbearing age EXCEPT
   1. prophylactic bed rest following a dural pressure
   2. direction of the needle bevel
   3. increased hydration
   4. use of pencil-point needles

Anesthesia for Obstetrics

Answers and Discussion

The authors have made every effort to thoroughly verify the answers to the questions that appear on the preceding pages. As in any text, however, some inaccuracies and ambiguities may occur. If in doubt, please consult the indicated reference. When no page number(s) are cited, the reference is to a journal article or to a refresher course lecture that should be read in its entirety.

The Editors

499. (C) Presentation is the relationship of the long axis of the fetus to the long axis of the mother. The fetal presentation may be longitudinal or transverse. With a longitudinal presentation the presenting part is either the head (cephalic) or the buttocks (breech). The shoulder is the presenting part with a transverse presentation. An oblique presentation is between the longitudinal and transverse. A cephalic presentation is classified according to the relationship of the fetal head to the fetal body (fetal attitude or habitus). This relationship depends on the degree of flexion or extension of the fetal head. The head may present as occiput (vertex), face, mentum (chin), sinciput (large fontanelle), or brow. A breech presentation is classified according to the flexion and extension of the thighs or knees. (**Ref. 34,** pp. 231–233)

500. (B) A breech presentation is the entrance of the fetal lower extremities or pelvis into the maternal pelvic inlet. A frank breech has hips flexed and knees extended. A complete breech has hips and knees flexed. An incomplete or footling breech has one or both hips extended and one or both feet below the buttocks. Breech presentation complicates 3% of deliveries, and the most common cause of breech presentation is prematurity. Other causes of breech presentation include uterine anomalies, fetal anomalies, multiple gestation, placenta previa, contracted maternal pelvis, and tumors obstructing the birth canal. (**Ref. 34, p. 689**)

501. (C) Fetal morbidity and mortality are higher in breech presentation than in cephalic presentation. One factor that contributes to the increased morbidity and mortality is birth asphyxia. Birth asphyxia can occur secondary to umbilical cord prolapse, arrest of the aftercoming head, or umbilical cord compression. Umbilical cord prolapse occurs in approximately 0.5% of cephalic presentations and 4% to 7% of breech presentations. The risk of cord prolapse with a frank breech approaches that of the cephalic presentation. Umbilical cord prolapse occurs in 4% to 5% of complete breeches and 10% of incomplete or footling breech presentations. (**Ref. 34, p. 689**)

502. (D) The goals of providing anesthesia for a vaginal breech delivery are adequate pain relief, prevention of a premature bearing-down reflex, maternal cooperation in a slow controlled delivery through a relaxed perineum, and the ability to relax the uterus rapidly if needed. There are three methods of a breech delivery: spontaneous, assisted, and total breech extraction. The entire infant delivers without any manipulation in a spontaneous breech delivery. In a partial breech extraction the infant is delivered spontaneously to the umbilicus, and then the obstetrician extracts the remainder of the body. The entire body of the infant is extracted in a total breech extraction. Forceps may be used to deliver the head in both partial and total breech extractions. (**Ref. 34, p. 691**)

503. (A) The pain of the first stage of labor is referred to the dermatomes supplied by the same spinal cord segments that receive input from the uterus and cervix. During the latent phase of the first stage of labor, pain is experienced as an ache and localized to the T_{11} and T_{12} dermatomes. Pain in the active phase incorporates T_{10} and L_1 and becomes localized to T_{10}, T_{11}, T_{12}, and L_1. The surface distribution over the back of the T_{10} through L_1 dermatomes overlies the lower three lumbar vertebrae and the upper half of the sacrum. The nature of the pain is described as visceral. (**Ref. 34**, pp. 256–257)

504. (B) Increasing pressure of the presenting part in the pelvis and the perineum becomes an additional source of pain in the second stage of labor. As the second stage progresses, there is additional distention of the subcutaneous tissues of the vagina that causes stretching and tearing of the fascia that result in pain. There is additional pain that results from stimulation of pain-sensitive structures within the pelvic cavity. These include traction on the pelvic parietal perineum and uterine ligaments; stretching and tension of the bladder, urethra, and rectum; stretching and tension of ligaments, fascia, and muscles of the pelvic cavity; and pressure on one or more roots of the lumbosacral plexus. Pain is transmitted via the spinal nerve roots, S_2, S_3, S_4 and is referred to the lower lumbar and sacral segments. The pain is typically well localized and somatic in nature. (**Ref. 34**, p. 258)

505. (A) The pudendal nerve is the peripheral nerve responsible for the transmission of pain from the lower vagina, vulva, and perineum. Distention of these areas produces pain during the second stage of labor. The pudendal nerve carries somatic nerves from the anterior primary divisions of the second, third, and fourth sacral nerves. Adequate bilateral pudendal nerve blockade, done at the completion of cervical dilatation, provides pain relief during the second stage of labor and delivery. Bilateral pudendal nerve block may also be used for vacuum or forceps deliveries and for repair of superficial to moderate vaginal and perineal lacerations. The most common local anesthetic used for bilateral pudendal nerve block is 1% lidocaine. The local anesthetic is injected near blood vessels. An intravascular injection with rapid systemic uptake can occur. Lidocaine is demonstrable in maternal and fetal blood within 5 min of the block, with peak concentrations occurring within 10 to 20 min. The most common maternal complication is inadequate analgesia secondary to performing the block too late after complete cervical dilatation. Other complica-

294 / 19: Anesthesia for Obstetrics

tions include systemic toxic reactions after an intravascular injection and too rapid absorption, or the administration of too much local anesthetic. Hematoma and subgluteal abscess formation have been reported. Fetal complications are rare and are primarily associated with fetal exposure to toxic amounts of local anesthetic. (**Ref. 34,** pp. 303–304)

506. **(D)** Pain during the first stage of labor is secondary to dilatation of the cervix and distention of the lower uterine segment. Pain fibers (Aδ and C fibers) from these structures converge on the paracervical plexus. A paracervical block diminishes pain during the first stage of labor by blocking afferent nerves at the paracervical or Frankenhauser's plexus. The plexus lies lateral and posterior to the uterine and cervical junction at the base of the broad ligament. The most serious complication of a paracervical block is fetal bradycardia. The mechanism of the fetal bradycardia is unclear. Mechanisms include direct transfer of local anesthesia across the placenta, a direct toxic affect on the fetal central nervous system and myocardium, decreased uteroplacental perfusion, and local anesthetic-induced uterine artery vasoconstriction. Bradycardia that lasts longer than 10 min can result in a transient fetal metabolic acidosis. The time for intrauterine resuscitation following transient bradycardia directly relates to neonatal outcome. Fetuses that are delivered 30 minutes or more after the transient bradycardic event have better Apgar scores. Should bradycardia occur following a paracervical block, all measures should be taken to optimize uteroplacental perfusion. Maternal complications are rare but include local anesthetic systemic toxicity, paracervical hematomas, vaginal lacerations, and, rarely, a subgluteal and retropsoas abscess. (**Ref. 34,** pp. 297–301)

507. **(A)** The first ligament encountered is the supraspinous. It connects the posterior borders of the spinous processes. The interspinous ligament connects the spines. The ligamentum flavum contains yellow elastic tissue and unites the inner surface of the lamina above, to the outer surface of the upper border of the lamina below. The ligamentum flavum is 3 to 5 mm thick. (**Ref. 34,** p. 309)

508. **(B)** Epidural opioids are most effective in reducing a visceral type of pain that characterizes the first stage of labor. Although

effective in reducing visceral type pain, epidural opioids are unpredictable as the sole analgesic agent for the first stage of labor. They are most effective in combination with dilute concentrations of local anesthetics. This combination can provide effective and reliable analgesia with a more rapid onset, more profound analgesia, less motor blockade, and longer duration of action than if local anesthetic or opioid were used alone. Epidural opioids alone have not been found to be effective in the treatment of the somatic type of pain that characterizes the second and third stages of labor. Opioids with greater lipid solubility have a more rapid uptake into the spinal cord, which results in a faster onset of analgesia. Morphine, which is hydrophilic, has an analgesia onset time from 15 to 60 min. On the other hand, fentanyl, sufentanyl, and alfentanyl, which are more lipid soluble, have an analgesia latency period of only 5 to 10 min. The more lipid soluble the opioid, the quicker the clearance and the shorter the duration of action. Hydrophilic opioids have a longer duration of action and rostral spread is characteristic. Peripheral nociceptors activate a thinly myelinated Aδ and unmyelinated C afferent nerve fibers. These pain fibers ultimately synapse with second-order neurons in the substantia gelatinosa of the dorsal horn as well as dendrites of deeper lying cells. Epidural opioids act to modulate the transmission of painful information through the μ receptor at the level of this synapse. (**Ref. 38,** pp. 158–162)

509. **(C)** 2-Chloroprocaine is the local anesthetic of choice for epidural anesthesia for cesarean section in the event of fetal distress. It rapidly produces intense motor and sensory blockade. It has a high therapeutic to toxic ratio and relatively large amounts of the drug can be administered quickly to achieve rapid onset. The drug is rapidly metabolized by plasma pseudocholinesterase and has a maternal serum half-life of approximately 40 seconds. Placental transfer is small, and fetal effects are negligible in the face of fetal acidosis. (**Ref. 34,** p. 327)

510. **(B)** The period of fetal development that is most susceptible to teratogenesis with exposure to anesthetic agents begins around days 15 to 18. This time coincides with the time when the primitive streak is established. This period of high susceptibility continues until day 30. After day 30, the susceptibility to teratogenic effects decreases until days 55 to 60, and the risk is minimal through day 90. Defects occur at later stages much less commonly. Different organs are susceptible at different times during this critical period of organogenesis. These include brain (days 18 to 38), heart (days 18 to 40), eyes (days 24 to 40), limbs (days 24 to 36), gonads (days 37 to 50), male genitalia (days 45 to 70), female genitalia (days 40 to 150). (**Ref. 6,** #265)

511. (**C**) Patients with a history of a prior low transverse cesarean section have a higher risk for the development of placenta previa in future pregnancies. Patients with a complete placenta previa who have a history of a previous low transverse cesarean section are predisposed to the development of a placenta accreta during pregnancy. Placenta previa refers to a situation in which the placenta is abnormally located within the uterus. A complete placenta previa refers to a placenta that entirely covers the internal cervical os. A placenta accreta refers to the situation in which the normal plane of division between the placenta and uterus is not present at the time of delivery of the placenta. Accreta refers to invasion of the placenta into the decidua basalis of the uterus. Placenta increta refers to invasion of the placenta into the myometrium, and placenta percreta refers to invasion of the placenta through the myometrium and across the uterine wall. Over 50% of term parturients with a placenta previa and one or more previous cesarean sections have been reported to subsequently undergo an obstetric hysterectomy for placenta accreta to control hemorrhage. In some institutions placenta accreta is the most frequent indication for an emergency obstetric hysterectomy. (**Ref. 6,** #412)

512. (**B**) The incidence of failed intubation in the obstetric population is approximately 1 in 280. This incidence is 8 times more frequent than in the general surgical patient population. An unhurried evaluation of all patients admitted into a labor and delivery unit can anticipate close to 90% of urgent or emergent cesarean deliveries. The anesthesiologist should use this time to identify the parturient who has a potentially difficult airway so that other health care personnel can be notified and management plans can be formulated. Part of the airway examination should include an attempt to visualize the normal oropharyngeal anatomy (soft palate, uvula, and tonsillar pillars). A patient whose oropharyngeal structures are partially or totally obliterated may have a glot-

tic opening that cannot be visualized. Obesity complicates a high percentage of anesthetic-related maternal deaths. Of these deaths, close to half involve general anesthesia for cesarean delivery. Fifty percent of the deaths associated with general anesthesia were directly due to failure to establish an adequate airway. The obese patient is at higher risk of requiring a cesarean delivery compared to the nonobese patient. (**Ref. 38**, pp. 475–481)

513. **(D)** The total blood volume is increased at term by 30% to 40% over the prepregnant state. There is a transfusion of 500 mL into the intravascular space with each contraction. Normal blood loss during an uncomplicated delivery is approximately 500 mL. During an uncomplicated caesarean section, or a twin delivery, the typical blood loss is in the range of 1,000 mL. The pregnant patient tolerates a blood loss of up to 1,500 mL because of the increase in total blood volume, autotransfusion of 500 mL at the time of delivery, and the decrease in vascular space with the contraction of the uterus after the delivery. (**Ref. 38**, p. 7)

514. **(B)** Pruritus is the most common side effect of intraspinal narcotics. The cause of the pruritus is unknown and does not appear to be related to histamine release. The onset occurs shortly after analgesia develops. The side effect is dose-related and as a result is more intense and occurs with a higher incidence with subarachnoid narcotics as compared to epidural narcotics. Treatment options include the administration of low dose naloxone, diphenhydramine (25 to 50 mg), or nalbuphine (10 mg subcutaneously). There may be an association between the use of intrathecal narcotics and the reactivation of oral herpes simplex virus. It has been suggested that patients with a history of herpes labialis should be warned of a possible reactivation. The incidence of mild to severe pruritus following epidural morphine has been reported in as many as 60%, with approximately 29% of patients requiring treatment. A 35% incidence of nausea and vomiting has been reported following epidural morphine, with up to 11% of patients requiring treatment. Treatment options include low-dose naloxone, metoclopramide (10 mg IV), droperidol (0.625 mg IV), and transdermal scopolamine patches. The incidence of urinary retention in the obstetric population is difficult to judge since the cesarean section patient, and often patients in labor, have an indwelling Foley catheter. Urinary retention occurs with the onset

of analgesia and may be mediated via detrusor muscle relaxation. The most serious side effect of intraspinal narcotics is delayed respiratory depression. This has occurred with both epidural and intrathecal narcotics and with both hydrophilic and lipid soluble agents. The reported incidence of respiratory depression with epidural opioids is 0.25% to 0.40% and approximately 4% to 7% with subarachnoid opiates. The respiratory depression has a biphasic pattern. The initial risk is within the first half hour after administration and represents elevated serum levels. The second peak of respiratory depression occurs approximately 4 to 8 hours after the epidural and is secondary to the rostral spread of narcotic in the CSF. The parturient should be monitored for side effects of epidural or intrathecal narcotics for 24 hours after administration. (**Ref. 38,** pp. 178–180)

515. **(B)** Abruptio placentae means the separation of a normally implanted placenta after 20 weeks' gestation and before birth of the fetus. The incidence varies from 0.2% to 2.4%. Maternal mortality is 1.8% to 2.8%, and perinatal mortality can be as high as 50%. Risk factors include hypertensive disorders, high parity, uterine abnormalities and a previous placental abruptio. The use of cocaine has been associated with abruptio placentae. The typical presentation is painful vaginal bleeding, associated with increased uterine activity and possibly fetal distress. The bleeding may be obvious (revealed hemorrhage) or may be concealed in the uteroplacental unit (internal or concealed hemorrhage). As a result, the amount of bleeding from abruptio placentae can be misleading and the amount of blood loss is commonly underestimated. Abruptio placentae can be classified as either mild, moderate, or severe. Mild or moderate abruptio is usually not associated with maternal hypotension, coagulopathy, or fetal distress. These account for about 85% to 90% of the abruptios. Severe abruptio (10% to 15%) is characterized by increased uterine activity, hypertension, maternal pain, fetal distress or fetal death, and coagulopathy. (**Ref. 38,** pp. 389–390)

516. **(C)** Oxygenated blood returns from the placenta to the fetus via the umbilical vein. Blood bypasses the liver by traversing the ductus venosus. Blood returning to the right side of the heart is preferentially shunted from the right atrium through the foramen ovale to the left atrium, then via the left ventricle to the fetal heart and brain. The shunting of blood from the ductus venosus to the left side of the circulation results in blood with the highest oxygen content perfusing organs that have the highest oxygen consumption, namely, the fetal heart and brain. (**Ref. 6,** #116)

517. (A) Prolonged duration of epidural anesthesia does not result in depressed neonates. Hypotension is common with regional anesthesia. If it is treated promptly, it does not result in low Apgar scores. Prolonged uterine incision to delivery time is directly related to fetal hypoxia and acidosis with either regional or general anesthesia. Uterine incision to delivery intervals exceeding 3 min are associated with a significantly lower pH and higher incidence of depressed Apgar scores in neonates. Unlike regional anesthesia, the duration of general anesthesia can influence neonatal outcome irrespective of the uterine incision to delivery time. The longer the duration of general anesthesia, the higher the incidence of neonatal depression. In one study, if the duration of exposure to general anesthesia was less than 5 min, 88% of neonates were given an Apgar score of 7 to 10. If the duration was 6 to 10 min, the percent fell to 74%; 11 to 20 min, 69%; 21 to 30 min, 50%; and if the duration of anesthesia was 31 to 60 min, the percent of neonates with Apgar scores between 7 to 10 fell to 36%. (**Ref. 38,** p. 237)

518. (A) Preeclampsia is the clinical triad of hypertension, proteinuria, and generalized edema occurring after 20 weeks' gestation. Hypertension is defined as an increase in the systolic and diastolic blood pressures of 30 and 15 mm of mercury respectively over baseline, a systolic blood pressure of at least 140 mm of mercury, or a diastolic blood pressure of at least 90 mm of mercury, or a mean blood pressure of at least 105 mm of mercury. Blood pressure measurement should be taken at least twice, six hours apart.

Proteinuria is defined as more than 300 mg per liter in a 24-hour collection or more than 1+ on a dip stick on two samples taken six hours apart.

Edema is defined as excess fluid in nondependent parts of the body.

Preeclampsia can be further defined as mild or severe. Mild preeclampsia includes a blood pressure of 140/90 or greater, proteinuria 1 to 2+ on dipstick or more than 300 mg in a 24-hour period but less than 5 g in a 24-hour period, and generalized edema. Severe preeclampsia is defined by a blood pressure of 160/110 or higher, proteinuria measured as 3 to 4+ on a dip stick, or more than 5 g in a 24-hour period reflecting renal damage, oliguria (less than 500 mL in a 24-hour period), CNS symptoms including visual disturbance or headache, right upper quadrant pain, evidence of pulmonary edema or cyanosis, or the diagnosis of the HELLP syndrome. (**Ref. 6,** #235)

519. (A) The intravascular volume of the preeclamptic patient is depleted. The plasma volume is estimated to be 300 to 500 mL less in the preeclamptic than the nonpreeclamptic pregnant patient. As a result the preeclamptic is relatively hemoconcentrated. There is a greater increase in plasma volume (50% to 55%) compared to red blood cell mass (30% to 50%) in the normal parturient. This results in a "physiologic anemia" of pregnancy (hemoglobin <11 g/dL). The preeclamptic frequently has a hematocrit above 35%. Mild to severe thrombocytopenia is common in preeclampsia, occurring 11% to 50% of the time. The etiology is an increase in peripheral consumption of platelets in association with endothelial cell injury. In addition to thrombocytopenia, preeclamptics may have altered platelet function. About 10% to 25% of preeclamptic patients with normal platelet counts (>100,000) have prolonged bleeding times (>10 minutes). The assessment of platelet function by bleeding time is currently controversial. It is debatable if the standardized bleeding time test reliably predicts the risk of bleeding in other areas of the body. There are no reports in the literature of a spontaneous epidural hematoma following the administration of epidural anesthesia to a preeclamptic patient. One must weigh the benefits of regional anesthesia with the risk of epidural hematoma when evaluating the coagulation status of the preeclamptic patient. (**Ref. 6,** #235)

520. (A) Upper airway edema is an expected physiologic change associated with pregnancy, but the edema can be markedly worse in preeclampsia and can lead to airway compromise. Thorough evaluation of the airway is essential in preeclampsia. Awake intubation and tracheostomy have been required in severe preeclampsia with extreme edema. A smaller size endotracheal tube (6.0) is recommended for the preeclamptic patient. One primary drug interaction to be considered when administering general anesthesia to the preeclamptic is the interaction of magnesium and muscle relaxants. The duration of action of depolarizing and nondepolarizing muscle relaxants can be prolonged in the face of elevated serum magnesium. Muscle relaxants should not be given following succinylcholine for intubation unless the response to nerve stimulation indicates the need to do so. Defasciculation with a nondepolarizer before the use of succinylcholine is usually unnecessary because magnesium blunts this response. Cerebral infarction is one of the leading causes of morbidity and mortality in these patients. Laryngoscopy and intubation, surgical stimulation, and emergence from general anesthesia can lead to significant increases in blood pressure, heart rate, and circulating catecholamines. Techniques to attenuate these responses in the preeclamptic patient should be determined prior to the induction of general anesthesia. Pharmacologic methods include the use of intravenous narcotics, lidocaine, and antihypertensive drugs. Various antihypertensive drugs including hydralazine, labetalol, trimethaphan, nitroglycerin, and nitroprusside have been used. Ketamine should be avoided in the preeclamptic patient because of its tendency to produce hypertension when administered in full anesthetic doses. Hydralazine has a slow unreliable response. Labetalol has a large variation in the effective dose and may not effectively lower blood pressure when used alone. Trimethaphan may interfere with pseudocholinesterase, resulting in a prolongation of succinylcholine. Nitroglycerin has a variable effect in the well-hydrated preeclamptic and can increase intracranial pressure. Nitroprusside may cause an increase in intracranial pressure and cyanide toxicity. The administration of esmolol to ewes has resulted in fetal hypoxemia, acidosis, and decreased heart rate. Human case reports cite significant fetal bradycardia with maternal administration. (**Ref. 38**, pp. 316–318, 320–322)

521. (C) The hemodynamic profile of the severely preeclamptic patient includes elevated systolic, diastolic, and mean arterial blood pressure, increased cardiac output, and normal or slightly increased systemic vascular resistance. The central venous pressure and pulmonary capillary wedge pressure may be low, normal, or high, and pulmonary capillary wedge pressure may not correlate in any given preeclamptic patient. Pulmonary vascular resistance is normal and colloid oncotic pressure is lower than in the normal pregnant patient. Colloid oncotic pressure correlates with decreased plasma protein levels in preeclamptics. Protein loss is via the kidney as well as through endothelial capillary leak. The decreased plasma oncotic pressure along with capillary endothelial damage may account for the majority of pulmonary edema that occurs in approximately 3% of the preeclamptic patients. 80% of the preeclamptic patients who develop pulmonary edema do so postpartum. (**Ref. 38,** pp. 309–311)

522. (D) The uterus of the preeclamptic patient is hyperactive and very sensitive to oxytocin. Induction is frequently successful and rapid labor is common. Preterm labor frequently occurs, and elective preterm delivery is often necessary for maternal indications. Prematurity significantly contributes to the increased perinatal morbidity and mortality in preeclampsia. Respiratory distress, intracranial hemorrhage, smallness for gestational age, and meconium aspiration contribute to the increased perinatal morbidity and mortality. Intervillous blood flow is decreased by 50% to 70% because of the increase in vascular resistance and increased maternal blood viscosity. The placenta is frequently small, infarcted, and shows evidence of premature aging. The incidence of abruptio is increased in both preeclampsia and eclampsia and in pregnancies complicated by hypertension from other causes. The number one cause of maternal death in preeclampsia/eclampsia is intracranial hemorrhage. (**Ref. 38,** p. 314)

523. (A) In the United States magnesium is currently the drug of choice for seizure prophylaxis in preeclampsia/eclampsia. The antiseizure activity is secondary to depression of the central nervous system. Magnesium is a mild vasodilator because of its depression of smooth muscle contraction and catecholamine release. However, its mild antihypertensive effects are unreliable and usually transient. The therapeutic serum concentration range of magnesium is 4.0 to 8.0 mEq per liter. It is associated with abnormal neuromuscular transmission in these dosages. It decreases the amount of acetylcholine released at the motor nerve terminals, decreases the sensitivity of the neuromuscular receptor at the motor endplate to the depolarizing action of acetylcholine, and decreases the excitability of the muscle membrane. Muscle weakness is possible, and elevated serum magnesium levels are associated with increased sensitivity of the patient to both depolarizing and nondepolarizing muscle relaxants. Respiratory insufficiency and cardiac failure can occur at serum levels that are associated with the loss of deep tendon reflexes. ECG changes can occur at

5.0 to 10 mEq per liter, specifically prolonged PQ interval and widened QRS complex. At 10 mEq per liter there may be a loss of deep tendon reflexes, at 15 mEq per liter sinoatrial and atrial ventricular block and respiratory paralysis, and at 25 mEq per liter cardiac arrest. Magnesium decreases uterine activity and is an effective tocolytic. It may produce uterine hypotonus at delivery. Magnesium does not appear to affect plasma cholinesterase activity or the metabolism of succinylcholine. It crosses the placenta but is not associated with significant negative side effects on the neonate at therapeutic levels. With higher levels the neonate may have decreased muscle tone, respiratory depression, and apnea. Magnesium undergoes renal elimination. Renal function must be evaluated prior to magnesium loading to determine the effective maintenance dose. (**Ref. 38,** pp. 315–316)

524. (A) Pregnant patients can desaturate quickly following succinylcholine-induced apnea. The greater fall in PO_2 in the pregnant patient is secondary to the decrease in functional residual capacity along with an increase in oxygen consumption. The supine position and general anesthesia augment the decrease in functional residual capacity. Adequate denitrogenation can occur with the pregnant patient breathing 100% oxygen for 3 min at a normal tidal volume or taking 4 breaths at vital capacity with 100% oxygen. (**Ref. 34,** pp. 14–15)

525. (B) Up to 15% of pregnant patients at term will experience a syndrome called *supine hypotension syndrome*. In this syndrome the inferior vena cava is totally obstructed by the gravid uterus when the patient assumes the supine position. Maternal symptoms are attributed to lack of venous return to the heart. Partial compression of the inferior vena cava is very common late in pregnancy before the presenting fetal part is fixed in the pelvis. This can lead to venous blood pooling and increased venous pressure in the lower extremities, which may explain the phlebitis and varicosities that can be found in the pregnant patient. Maintaining left uterine displacement or turning the pregnant patient completely on her left side can relieve the obstruction. Obstruction of the inferior vena cava can lead to an increase in uterine venous pressure. This may affect uterine perfusion since uterine blood flow is directly related to the perfusion pressure. Compression of the aorta by the gravid uterus is less common but can occur. It is not associated with maternal symptoms but can cause a decrease in blood flow to the lower extremities and uterine arteries. The latter can lead to a decrease in uterine blood flow. Aortocaval compression can aggravate potential hypotensive side effects of those anesthetic drugs that cause vasodilation, as well as techniques that cause sympathetic blockade such as subarachnoid and epidural block. As a result, arterial hypotension is more common and severe during anesthesia in pregnancy when compared to the nonpregnant patient. The pregnant patient at term should not be allowed to assume the supine position. Prevention of aortocaval compression is possible with left uterine displacement. (**Ref. 34,** pp. 6–7)

526. (E) Total blood volume increases 35% to 40% above prepregnant levels. The increase in total blood volume is secondary to an increase in both plasma and volume of red blood cells, although the plasma volume increases to a greater extent than the red blood cell volume and results in a physiologic anemia of pregnancy. A normal hematocrit in the parturient is 33% to 35%. Cardiac output increases 40% over prepregnant levels, increases further during labor, and reaches its highest level immediately postpartum when cardiac output may be 80% greater than the prepregnant levels. Total peripheral resistance falls by approximately 15% and results in a decrease in maternal blood pressure. Systolic blood pressure can range from 0 to 15 mm Hg and diastolic blood pressure can range anywhere from 10 to 20 mm Hg below prepregnant values. Central venous pressure and pulmonary capillary wedge pressure are normal in pregnancy despite the increase in total blood volume. (**Ref. 34,** pp. 6–9)

527. (D) All pregnant patients are considered to have full stomachs and be at risk for acid aspiration regardless of the time the patient has been NPO. Fatal aspiration is eight times more likely in the pregnant patient than in the nonpregnant patient. Gastric emptying is prolonged and gastric pH is reduced. The latter is secondary to the production of placental gastrin, which raises the acid, chloride, and enzyme content of the stomach. In addition, the gravid uterus alters the angle of the gastroesophageal junction that results in incompetence of the junction and predisposes the pregnant patient to reflux, heartburn, and silent regurgitation. In addition, pain and narcotics can delay gastric emptying time. Unless there is an absolute contraindication, all patients should undergo rapid sequence induction with cricoid pressure for the administration of general anesthesia. Only nonparticulate antacids should be administered to the parturient prior to the administration of a general anesthetic. Aspiration of a particulate antacid, such as Mylanta or Maalox, can cause a severe aspiration pneumonitis. All patients should receive a nonparticulate antacid prior to the administration of general anesthesia. If time permits, an H_2 blocker or metoclopramide is considered safe to use in pregnancy. (**Ref. 38,** pp. 414, 417–418)

528. (**C**) Adjusting the pH of local anesthetic solutions to a more alkaline level converts more of the molecule into the nonionized lipid-soluble form. This is because local anesthetics are basic molecules, all with PKAs greater than 7.4. A more alkaline environment results in a higher proportion of the molecule existing in the lipid soluble nonionized form. This nonionized form can readily cross the cellular membrane to bind to the sodium–potassium receptor channels. The pH adjustment of lidocaine has been shown to decrease onset time. It remains controversial if the pH adjustment of chloroprocaine significantly decreases onset time. The pH adjustment of bupivicaine is problematic because of a narrow margin between satisfactory alkalinization and precipitation of the base. (**Ref. 38,** p. 91)

529. (**B**) Although there is a wide range of reported incidences of headache among various investigators using the same size needle, all investigators would agree that a smaller needle is less likely to result in a postdural puncture headache. When using a needle with a beveled tip, placing the bevel parallel to the longitudinal fibers of the dura lowers the incidence of headache. A parallel insertion of the needle bevel through the dura probably minimizes the size of the dural hole. The use of pencil point needles, such as Whitaker or Sprotte needles, spread rather than cut dural fibers. Spread is associated with a significantly lower incidence of a postdural puncture headache. Bedrest for 24 hours following a dural puncture has not been shown to decrease the incidence of development of a spinal headache nor has hydration following dural puncture affected the incidence of a subsequent headache. (**Ref. 34,** pp. 768–772)

20

Anesthesia for Pediatric Surgery

DIRECTIONS (Questions 530–549): Each of the questions or incomplete statements below is followed by five suggested answers or completions. Select the **one** that is best in each case.

530. What is the normal volume of blood in a normal, healthy term infant?
   A. 65 mL/kg
   B. 75 mL/kg
   C. 85 mL/kg
   D. 100 mL/kg
   E. 125 mL/kg

531. A 12-kg, one-year-old infant is undergoing an emergency laparotomy for intussusception. He has had an IV in place for one day and has a good urine output. What should the rate of infusion be during the surgical procedure?
   A. 60 mL/hr
   B. 80 mL/hr

C. 100 mL/hr
D. 120 mL/hr
E. 160 mL/hr

532. A two-year-old presenting for elective repair of a bilateral inguinal hernia must be NPO how long before surgery?
    A. 3 hr for clear liquids, 4 hr for solids
    B. 2 hr for clear liquids, 6 hr for solids
    C. 3 hr for clear liquids, 8 hr for solids
    D. 3 hr for clear liquids, 6 hr for solids
    E. 2 hr for clear liquids, 4 hr for solids

533. A three-month-old male child has pyloric stenosis. He has been vomiting for three days and has a sunken fontanelle, tachycardia, poor skin turgor, and oliguria. The severity of his dehydration, expressed in percentage is
    A. 3%
    B. 5%
    C. 10%
    D. 15%
    E. 20%

534. Regarding the patient in question 533, which of the following statements is true?
    A. rehydrate patient and operate immediately
    B. the serum sodium and chloride would be normal
    C. metabolic alkalosis with hyperchloremia is present
    D. hyponatremia and hypochloremia are present
    E. the patient has a severe metabolic acidosis

535. Which of the following statements about neonatal temperature regulation is NOT true?
    A. brown fat is a major source of thermogenesis
    B. the anterior hypothalamus responds to cold, the posterior hypothalamus responds to heat
    C. heat loss from an uncovered head can account for up to 60% of total heat loss
    D. temperature receptors are located in the skin, the CNS, and the GI tract
    E. temperature receptors are more sensitive to rapid changes than to gradual ones

308 / 20: Anesthesia for Pediatric Surgery

536. Risk factors for retinopathy of prematurity (ROP) include all the following EXCEPT
  A. prematurity
  B. prolonged exposure to high O_2 concentrations
  C. intracranial hemorrhage
  D. septicemia
  E. patent ductus arteriosus (PDA)

537. When comparing an adult airway to that of a newborn, which of the following statements is FALSE?
  A. adults' vocal folds have a lower anterior than posterior attachment to the glottis
  B. newborns have large heads relative to their bodies
  C. a newborn's larynx is high in the neck (C_{3-4} compared to C_{4-5} in adults)
  D. the narrowest portion of the newborn's airway is at the cricoid ring
  E. glossoptosis is abnormal in both adults and children

538. All the following statements regarding the laryngeal mask airway are true EXCEPT
  A. it can be used in patients with full stomachs
  B. if of proper size, one cannot intubate the trachea of the patient
  C. proper positioning is ascertained by end-tidal carbon dioxide tracing and bilateral breath sounds
  D. if the mask is rotated, total airway obstruction may occur
  E. the mask can be used as an aid in the management of a difficult airway

539. The features found in the Treacher–Collins syndrome include the following EXCEPT
  A. mandibular hypoplasia
  B. abnormal ear shapes
  C. hemifacial microsomia
  D. congenital heart disease
  E. downward-sloping palpebral fissures

540. Which heart defect is most commonly seen in children with Down syndrome (trisomy 21)?
  A. ventricular septal defect (VSD)
  B. atrioventricular septal defect (AVSD)
  C. atrial septal defect (ASD)
  D. tetralogy of Fallot (TOF)
  E. transposition of the great arteries (TGA)

541. The most common form of tracheoesophageal fistula is
  A. esophageal atresia; upper segment of the esophagus communicates with the trachea
  B. esophageal atresia; lower segment of the esophagus communicates with the trachea
  C. esophageal atresia; both upper and lower segments of the esophagus communicate with the trachea
  D. no esophageal atresia but communication somewhere with the trachea
  E. no esophageal atresia but communication with the right mainstem bronchus

542. All the following statements regarding the transitional circulation in the newborn are true EXCEPT
  A. the complete transition from fetal to adult circulation does not occur at the time of birth only
  B. pulmonary vascular resistance decreases by 75% with the newborn's first breath
  C. fetal circulation is a circuit in parallel
  D. blood can shunt through a patent ductus arteriosus
  E. prostaglandin E_1 contracts the ductus arteriosus

310 / 20: Anesthesia for Pediatric Surgery

543. Which of the following statements is true regarding newborn cardiovascular physiology?
   A. the newborn myocardium is less sensitive to the cardiac depressant effects of halothane
   B. a newborn has a very well-developed sympathetic nervous system
   C. when faced with falling cardiac output, the newborn will usually increase stroke volume
   D. a newborn has a very well-developed parasympathetic nervous system
   E. the neonate has a very compliant myocardium

544. You are evaluating your patient the night before surgery. When you arrive in the room, a two-year-old 15-kg boy with uncorrected tetralogy of Fallot develops a "tet spell." Which of the following therapeutic maneuvers would NOT be indicated? (02 sat 65%, HR 70)
   A. administer 10 μg of IV isoproterenol
   B. administer O_2 by mask
   C. place the child in a "knee–chest" position
   D. administer 10 μg of phenylephrine IV
   E. administer 1.0 mg $MgSO_4$ IV

545. The earliest clinically evident sign or symptom of malignant hyperthermia is
   A. cardiac arrhythmias
   B. muscle rigidity
   C. cyanosis
   D. hyperthermia
   E. tachycardia and tachypnea

546. A premature infant is
   A. less than 35 weeks' gestation
   B. less than 37 weeks' gestation
   C. usually small for gestational age (SGA)
   D. usually intrauterine growth retarded (IUGR)
   E. usually large for gestational age (LGA)

547. A premature infant is at greatest risk for the apnea of prematurity at or below what postconceptual age?
  A. 40 weeks
  B. 45 weeks
  C. 50 weeks
  D. 55 weeks
  E. 60 weeks

548. The ideal endotracheal tube size for a four-year-old child is
  A. 3.5
  B. 4.0
  C. 4.5
  D. 5.0
  E. 5.5

549. A two-year-old male with a full stomach presents with epiglottitis. Ideal management for this child includes
  A. IV induction without muscle relaxants
  B. awake intubation
  C. inhalational induction with muscle relaxants
  D. IV induction with muscle relaxants
  E. inhalational induction without muscle relaxants

DIRECTIONS (Questions 550–565): For each of the questions or incomplete answers below, one or more of the answers or completions are correct. Select
  A. if only 1, 2, and 3 are correct
  B. if only 1 and 3 are correct
  C. if only 2 and 4 are correct
  D. if only 4 is correct
  E. if all are correct

---

550. Infants with prolonged vomiting from pyloric stenosis become hypokalemic due to
  1. loss of K^+ in vomitus
  2. K^+ shifts intracellularly due to metabolic alkalosis
  3. exchange of H^+ ions for K^+ ions in renal tubules
  4. lack of dietary intake

551. An anesthetized three-month-old male is lying on the operating room table. The room temperature is 76°F (24.4°C). The baby is naked and uncovered. Heat loss is due to
    1. conduction
    2. convection
    3. radiation
    4. evaporation

552. When comparing the adult O_2–Hb dissociation curve to that of the newborn
    1. fetal Hb has a higher affinity for O_2 than adult Hb
    2. 2–3 DPG interacts with Hb to increase O_2 affinity
    3. the P_{50} of fetal Hb is 18 torr
    4. the newborn O_2–Hb dissociation curve shifts to right

553. Which of the following statements is true about cuffed endotracheal tubes?
    1. they are required in adults because larynx has an irregular shape
    2. they can be used in children older than 8 years
    3. cuffed tubes are not advisable in small children because the volume of the cuff requires that a smaller ET tube be used
    4. N_2O can diffuse into an inflatable cuff

554. A three-year-old male presents to the ER with stridor. Which of the following symptoms would be associated with epiglottitis?
    1. "steeple sign" on AP view of neck
    2. barking cough
    3. inspiratory stridor
    4. drooling

555. Which of the following symptoms have been associated with Down syndrome (trisomy 21)?
    1. macroglossia
    2. hypothyroidism
    3. congenital heart disease
    4. leukemia

556. Which of the following statement(s) is (are) true regarding neonatal versus adult work of breathing?
1. nasal passages account for 50% of the total resistance to airflow in the neonate
2. in adults, the small airways provide the major proportion of airways resistance
3. O_2 consumption in the neonate is five times that of an adult
4. neonates have fewer type I muscle fibers present in the intercostal muscles and the diaphragm

557. Metaproterenol (alupent)
1. is a beta$_1$ sympathomimetic agent
2. is a beta$_2$ sympathomimetic agent
3. is a phosphodiasterase inhibitor
4. alters the c-AMP/c-GMP ratios

558. Which of the following statements is true for a newborn with an omphalocele?
1. it is associated with other congenital anomalies
2. it is periumbilical
3. it is due to a failure of the gut to migrate from the yolk sac into the abdomen
4. it is always exposed to air immediately after birth

559. Tetralogy of Fallot is a congenital heart lesion with anatomical defects that include
1. overriding aorta
2. L to R shunting through a VSD
3. pulmonary stenosis
4. hypoplastic left ventricle

560. Children with hypoplastic left heart syndrome
1. have absent left sided forces on ECG
2. are dependent on a patent ductus arteriosus for early survival
3. are candidates for the Norwood procedure
4. are candidates for the arterial switch procedure

561. Which of the following statement(s) is (are) true in regard to the autonomic nervous system in the newborn?
   1. the sympathetic nervous system is well developed
   2. the parasympathetic nervous system is well developed
   3. peripheral vascular resistance is high
   4. vagal tone is high

562. The MAC of halothane in a six-month-old child is
   1. 1.2%
   2. greater than in an adult
   3. greater than in a newborn
   4. less than in an adult

563. Which of the following situations puts a newborn at risk for neonatal hypoglycemia?
   1. prematurity
   2. maternal diabetes
   3. preeclampsia
   4. Beckwith Wiedemann syndrome

564. Which of the following symptoms is associated with Beckwith Wiedemann syndrome?
   1. macroglossia
   2. neonatal hypoglycemia
   3. omphalocele
   4. retrognathia

565. With regard to muscle relaxants
   1. neonates are less sensitive to the effects of nondepolarizing muscle relaxants than adults
   2. neonates are less sensitive to the effects of depolarizing muscle relaxants than adults
   3. neonates are more sensitive to the effects of depolarizing muscle relaxants than adults
   4. neonates are more sensitive to the effects of nondepolarizing muscle relaxants than adults

Anesthesia for Pediatric Surgery

Answers and Discussion

The authors have made every effort to thoroughly verify the answers to the questions that appear on the preceding pages. As in any text, however, some inaccuracies and ambiguities may occur. If in doubt, please consult the indicated reference. When no page number(s) are cited, the reference is to a journal article or to a refresher course lecture that should be read in its entirety.

The Editors

530. (C) The normal blood volume of a term newborn is 80 to 85 mL/kg. This decreases with age. The blood volumes in this age group are as follows:

Preemies 90 to 100 mL/kg
Neonates 80 to 85 mL/kg
Infants 80 mL/kg
Older children 60 to 75 mL/kg

(**Ref. 19,** p. 1277)

531. (E) The intraoperative fluid requirements are calculated by adding the maintenance fluid requirements (insensible loss due to metabolism, fluid lost from the respiratory tract, and urine output), fluid deficit (NPO time, loss from preoperative bleeding, and diarrhea and/or vomiting), and intraoperative fluid loss. The total intraoperative fluids required for this child are 164 mL/hr. This is calculated as follows:

10 mL/kg/hr for abdominal surgery (10 × 12 = 120 mL) maintenance fluids: 4 mL/kg/hr for 1st 10 kg
2mL/kg/hr for 2nd 10 kg; 1mL/kg/hr for anything over 20 kg.
(Ref. 19, p. 585)

532. **(D)** The current fasting guidelines for surgery are as follows:

Age	Fasting Time	
	Clear Liquids	Solids
< 6 mo	2 hr	4 hr
6 to 36 mo	3 hr	6 hr
>36 mo	3 hr	8 hr

(**Ref. 10,** pp. 176–177)

533. **(C)** The relationship of the physical findings to the severity of the dehydration in children is as follows:

Physical Findings	% of dehydration
Poor tissue turgor, dry mouth	5
Sunken fontanelle, tachycardia, oliguria	10
Sunken eyeballs, hypotension	15
Coma	20

(**Ref. 10,** p. 177)

534. **(D)** The classic findings in children with pyloric stenosis include dehydration, metabolic alkalosis, hyponatremia, and hypochloremia. Pyloric stenosis is not a surgical emergency. Children with metabolic derangements should be stabilized before surgery. (**Ref. 19,** pp. 602–603)

535. **(B)** Because an infant is unable to shiver, a newborn will respond to hypothermia by nonshivering thermogenesis. This is accomplished by metabolizing brown fat, which is located in the infant's mediastinum, and behind the scapulae. Heat loss from an

uncovered head can account for up to 60% of the total heat loss in an infant. Temperature receptors are located in the skin, GI tract, and CNS. In both adults and children, the anterior hypothalamus responds to heat, and the posterior hypothalamus responds to cold. (**Ref. 10,** pp. 31–37)

536. (**C**) Prematurity, exposure to high inspired FiO_2, septicemia, the presence of a patent ductus arteriosus, and Vitamin E deficiency have all been implicated in the development of the retinopathy of prematurity. There is no correlation, however, between the development or presence of intracranial hemorrhage and the retinopathy of prematurity. (**Ref. 39,** pp. 640–641)

537. (**A**) A newborn's vocal folds have a lower attachment to the glottis anteriorly than posteriorly, whereas the adult vocal folds are perpendicular to the axis of the trachea. Glossoptosis (abnormal at any age) is defined as the downward and backward displacement of the tongue toward the posterior pharyngeal wall. (**Ref. 10,** pp. 55–83)

538. (**A**) The LMA can be used to maintain airway patency in both difficult and routine airways. It can also be used as an obturator to place an endotracheal tube. Because it is seated outside the glottis, endobronchial intubation cannot occur if properly sized. Even though properly inserted, rotation can lead to total airway obstruction. The LMA is contraindicated in patients with a full stomach. (**Ref. 7,** pp. 688–689)

539. (**C**) The features of the Treacher Collins syndrome include mandibular and malar hypoplasia, retrognathia, micrognathia, abnormal ear shapes, congenital heart disease, downward-sloping palpebral fissures, but normal intelligence. Hemifacial microsomia is a feature of the Goldenhar's syndrome, not of the Treacher Collins syndrome. (**Ref. 19,** p. 1170)

540. (**B**) Almost 50% of children with Down syndrome have congenital heart disease, with an atrial-ventricular septal defect (AVSD) or endocardial cushion defect being the most common. Features common to these cardiac defects include a common AV valve, with potential for incompetence, and variable size defects in both the atrial and ventricular septa. Blood usually shunts from left to right in this defect, from the LV to the RA. This will lead to RA and RV volume overload and result in CHF if left untreated. (**Ref. 40,** pp. 842–843)

541. **(B)** The most common form of TE fistula is esophageal atresia with a distal fistula, seen in 80% to 90% of all cases. The presenting signs and symptoms of a TEF are polyhydramnios, early feeding difficulties (e.g., choking, regurgitation, aspiration), increased oronasal secretions, and abdominal distention. Preoperative evaluation of children with a TEF should include a careful investigation for other congenital anomalies, especially cardiac ones, since they may affect survival. (**Ref. 19,** p. 921)

542. **(E)** The transition from fetal to adult circulation begins at birth with the newborn's first breath but does not become complete for several days. With that first breath, a newborn's pulmonary vascular resistance drops by 75%. Blood can be shunted from left to right, both through a patent foramen ovale (atrial septum) and through a patent ductus arteriosus. Prostaglandins E_1 and E_2 (PGE_1, PGE_2) have been shown to relax the ductus arteriosus. (**Ref. 10,** pp. 272–275)

543. **(D)** The newborn's myocardium is poorly compliant. It is more sensitive to the myocardial depressant effects of volatile anesthetics and is more dependent on heart rate than stroke volume to increase cardiac output. The sympathetic nervous system is poorly developed in the newborn, whereas the parasympathetic nervous system is fully developed at birth. (**Ref. 10,** pp. 275–276)

544. **(A)** "Tet spells" are thought to be due in part to a spasm of the infundibular region below the pulmonary valve, which further increases the right-to-left shunting across a VSD. Some patients may benefit from propanolol (a beta-blocker). Isuprel, a beta-agonist, may make the "Tet spell" worse by potentiating the infundibular spasm. (**Ref. 28,** p. 245)

545. **(E)** Malignant hyperthermia (MH) is characterized by hypermetabolism. Its signs and symptoms include cardiac arrhythmias, trismus, muscle rigidity, hyperthermia, cyanosis, increase in PCO_2 and $ETCO_2$, metabolic and respiratory acidosis, increased serum lactate and increased urine and serum CPK. The earliest clinically

evident signs of MH, however, are tachycardia and tachypnea. (**Ref. 10**, pp. 427–428)

546. **(B)** By definition a premature infant is a neonate born before 37 weeks of gestation. A newborn may be SGA (small for gestational age), LGA (large for gestational age), or IUGR (intrauterine growth retarded), and still not be premature. (**Ref. 10**, p. 8)

547. **(B)** Postconceptual age (PCA) equals gestational age (GA) plus age after birth. Because the greatest risk for apnea of prematurity following anesthesia occurs in premature infants who are 50 weeks postconceptual age or less, it is important to remember that when a child who is 50 weeks or less PCA is admitted postoperatively to the PACU and hence to the NICU, the infant's cardiorespiratory status must be monitored continuously. (**Ref. 10**, p. 8)

548. **(D)** The formula for ET tube size (inner diameter) in children is:

$$\frac{Age + 16}{4}$$

In spite of this largely reliable formula, it is prudent to have three sizes of tube available in all cases—the calculated size, one size smaller, and one size larger than calculated from the formula. (**Ref. 10**, p. 69)

549. **(E)** The ideal management for a child with a full stomach and epiglottitis is an inhalation induction without the use of muscle relaxants. Under no circumstances should a child like this be examined in the office or emergency room. The first examination of the mouth or pharynx should be done in the operating room, with the surgeon standing by prepared to do an emergency cricothyrotomy. (**Ref. 10**, pp. 251–253)

550. **(A)** Infants with prolonged vomiting from pyloric stenosis become hypokalemic due to an intracellular shift of K^+, secondary to metabolic alkalosis, and loss of K^+ in urine and vomitus. Another electrolyte abnormality commonly seen in children with pyloric stenosis is a hypochloremic metabolic alkalosis. This is due to the loss of HCl in the infant's vomitus. (**Ref. 19**, pp. 602–603)

320 / 20: Anesthesia for Pediatric Surgery

551. (E) Because an infant has a much greater ratio of body surface area to weight than an adult, heat loss can occur much more rapidly. When heat is lost from this patient, it is lost via the following physical mechanisms: (1) conduction, or the transfer heat from the baby to the bed; (2) convection, which occurs when cold room air circulating around the infant removes a layer of heated air just above the skin; (3) radiation—in the absence of a radiant heat lamp, heat from the infant radiates to the cold wall; and (4) evaporation of water through skin and lungs. (**Ref. 10,** pp. 31–37)

552. (B) Fetal hemoglobin has a much higher affinity for oxygen than does adult hemoglobin. Since the P_{50} (partial pressure of O_2 when Hb is 50% saturated) is much less with fetal Hb when compared to that of an adult (18 torr versus 27 torr), fetal Hb gives up less O_2 to the tissues than adult Hb does. Therefore, the newborn oxygen–hemoglobin dissociation curve is shifted to the left, and 2–3 DPG interacts with Hb to decrease O_2 affinity. This shifts the O_2–Hb dissociation curve to the right, decreasing the hemoglobin's affinity for O_2. (**Ref. 19,** p. 33)

553. (E) The narrowest portion of the immature airway is at the level of the cricoid ring, and it is circular in shape. The shape of the ET tube therefore approximates the shape of the airway, allowing for a good seal. (**Ref. 19,** p. 464)

554. (D) Children with epiglottitis, present with a sudden onset of high fever, muffled voice, drooling, severe sore throat, and a positive "thumb sign" on lateral neck x-rays. Children with croup (laryngotracheal bronchitis; i.e., LTB) have a more gradual onset, barking cough, inspiratory stridor, and the "steeple sign" on AP views of the neck. (**Ref. 10,** pp. 251–255)

555. (E) Children with Down syndrome (trisomy 21) can present with a variety of symptoms, both anatomic and metabolic. Macroglossia and mental retardation are seen in 100% of Down children. Congenital heart disease occurs in up to 50% of the affected individuals, and subluxation of C_1–C_2 can be seen in 15% of these patients over the age of two years. Hypothyroidism and leukemia have been reported in infancy. (**Ref. 40,** pp. 842–843)

556. (D) Type I muscle fibers permit prolonged repetitive movement. Neonates have fewer Type I muscle fibers than do adults. Nasal passages account for 25% of the total airway resistance to airflow in the neonate. The nasal passages provide the major proportion of airway resistance in the adult, compared to small airways providing the major proportion of airway resistance in neonates. O_2 consumption in the neonate is only twice that of the adult. (**Ref. 10,** p. 64)

557. (C) Drugs that alter the c-AMP/c-GMP ratio are the β_2 sympathomimetic agents (metaproterenol, albuterol, isoetharine, and aminophylline (a phosphodiesterase inhibitor). (**Ref. 15,** pp. 110–111, 204; **Ref. 19,** pp. 937–938)

558. (B) Omphaloceles are caused by the failure of the gut to migrate early in gestation and is, therefore, frequently associated with other congenital anomalies. They are covered with a membrane at birth and are always midline. Gastroschisis is due to the occlusion of the omphalomesenteric artery, which occurs later in pregnancy and is usually an isolated finding. They are never covered with a membrane and are always periumbilical. (**Ref. 10,** pp. 240–242)

559. (B) Beyond the newborn period, Tetralogy of Fallot (TOF) is the most common form of cyanotic heart disease. TOF consists of a complex including a VSD, overriding aorta (the aortic valve straddles the ventricular septum), pulmonary stenosis, and right ventricular hypertrophy. Because of pulmonary outflow tract obstruction, blood is shunted from right to left, across the VSD, bypassing the lungs and leading to cyanosis. (**Ref. 28,** pp. 243–252)

560. (A) Children with hypoplastic left heart syndrome (HLHS) have small or atretic mitral and aortic valves, and a diminutive left ventricle. This leads to absent left-sided manifestations on the ECG. Since no functional left ventricle exists, the right ventricle in these children must perfuse the body through a patent ductus arterosus (PDA). The current treatment options for children with HLHS are (1) do nothing (100% mortality rate), (2) neonatal heart transplant, or (3) the Norwood procedure. The arterial switch procedure is indicated for children with transposition of the great arteries. (**Ref. 28,** pp. 271–273)

322 / 20: Anesthesia for Pediatric Surgery

561. **(C)** Peripheral vascular resistance is low in the newborn period because the sympathetic nervous system is poorly developed at birth but continues to develop postnatally. Vagal tone is high at birth because the parasympathetic nervous system is fully developed. (**Ref. 10,** p. 276)

562. **(A)** The MAC of halothane in a newborn is 0.87%, rising to a peak of 1.2% at 6 months of age before gradually falling to the adult level of 0.76%. (**Ref. 19,** p. 563)

563. **(E)** Term infants, less than 72 hours of age, with whole blood glucose levels of less than 40 mg/dL are considered to be suffering from hypoglycemia. Neonates at risk for hypoglycemia include preterm infants, infants of diabetic mothers (IDM), infants of preeclamptic mothers, infants in fetal distress, and infants with the Beckwith Wiedemann syndrome. (**Ref. 19,** p. 242)

564. **(A)** The Beckwith Wiedemann syndrome is a congenital disease of the newborn with physical findings that include macroglossia (leading to difficult intubation), omphalocele, organomegaly, neonatal hypoglycemia, and hypocalcemia. (**Ref. 10,** p. 81)

565. **(C)** Compared to adults, neonates are less sensitive to the effects of depolarizing muscle relaxants and more sensitive to the effects of nondepolarizing muscle relaxants. (**Ref. 19,** pp. 401–405)

21
Intensive Care Unit

DIRECTIONS (Questions 566–578): Each of the questions or incomplete statements below is followed by five suggested answers or completions. Select the **one** that is best in each case.

566. Treatment of status asthmaticus may include
    A. fluid restriction
    B. β_1 adrenergic agonists
    C. α adrenergic agonists
    D. inhaled ipratroprium bromide
    E. a reduced infusion rate of theophylline in smokers

567. In the adult respiratory distress syndrome (ARDS)
    A. alveolar edema occurs as a result of increased pulmonary capillary hydrostatic pressure
    B. lung compliance is increased
    C. pancreatitis may be the cause
    D. the etiology of the pulmonary failure is identified by examination of the chest x-ray
    E. positive end expiratory pressure (PEEP) can be used to increase intrapulmonary shunt

568. When an intra-aortic balloon pump is being used
   A. after balloon deflation the assisted systole is increased compared to unassisted systole
   B. cardiac function is improved by an increase in preload to the left ventricle by balloon inflation
   C. blood pressure is increased through an increase in afterload during systole
   D. coronary blood flow is increased by balloon inflation during diastole
   E. balloon inflation should be timed to occur at the same time as aortic valve opening

569. Characteristic hemodynamic changes of early septic shock include
   A. bradycardia
   B. low systemic vascular resistance
   C. high pulmonary capillary wedge pressure
   D. low cardiac output
   E. low mixed venous oxygen saturation (SvO_2)

570. Oxygen delivery to the tissues (DO_2) is increased by
   A. anemia
   B. increased oxygen consumption by the tissues
   C. hypoxia
   D. hypovolemia
   E. increased cardiac output

571. Arterial lines
   A. should be avoided in the ulnar artery because it is an end artery
   B. do not cause catheter-related sepsis
   C. may be inserted in the femoral artery if there is no significant atherosclerosis of the vessel
   D. may produce an incorrectly low mean blood pressure if the wave form is overdamped
   E. are less accurate than a blood pressure cuff for measuring BP in critically ill patients

572. In the fat embolism syndrome
   A. operative immobilization of the fracture should be delayed if the patient has respiratory distress
   B. a petechial rash develops on the trunk, which blanches under pressure
   C. cerebral involvement is unusual
   D. fat globules may be identified in the sputum
   E. the syndrome occurs at the time of the injury

573. Which of the following is compatible with the diagnosis of irreversible brain stem death?
   A. temperature less than 30°C
   B. seizure activity
   C. spinal reflexes
   D. unknown cause of coma
   E. decerebrate posturing

574. Amrinone
   A. has $beta_1$ adrenergic agonist activity
   B. may cause thrombocytopenia with prolonged administration
   C. causes vasoconstriction as the dose is increased
   D. is a potent antiarrhythmic agent
   E. decreases the amount of intracellular cyclic adenosine monophosphate (cAMP)

575. With regard to the arrhythmias
   A. a wide complex tachycardia may be supraventricular in origin
   B. amiodarone may be used to treat supraventricular and ventricular tachycardias
   C. lidocaine is indicated for supraventricular tachycardias
   D. procainamide is indicated for Torsade de Pointes ventricular tachycardia
   E. first-degree AV block is defined by a P–R interval greater than 0.12 seconds

576. Acute delirium occurring in the intensive care unit
   A. is usually due to preexisting psychiatric disorders
   B. should not be treated with haloperidol because of the risk of extrapyramidal side effects
   C. is less common in the elderly
   D. may result in a disturbed sleep-wake cycle
   E. may be improved by amitriptyline

577. Pseudomembranous colitis
   A. is caused by *Clostridium welchii*
   B. may be caused by vancomycin
   C. is a variant of Crohn's disease
   D. may be treated with clindamycin
   E. presents with watery diarrhea

578. In regard to the dialysis techniques
   A. continuous arteriovenous hemofiltration (CAVH) is inefficient for the removal of fluid
   B. hemodialysis is the method of choice for a cardiovascularly unstable patient
   C. peritoneal dialysis carries a risk of peritonitis
   D. CAVH does not require anticoagulation
   E. short periods of peritoneal dialysis are more efficient than hemodialysis

---

DIRECTIONS (Questions 579–598): For each of the questions or incomplete answers below, **one** or **more** of the answers or completions are correct. Select
   A. if only 1, 2, and 3 are correct
   B. if only 1 and 3 are correct
   C. if only 2 and 4 are correct
   D. if only 4 is correct
   E. if all are correct

---

579. During weaning from ventilation
   1. inadequate nutrition may reduce the ability to wean
   2. excess nutrition may reduce the ability to wean

3. the appearance of hypercapnia may be due to respiratory muscle weakness
4. a maximum inspiratory pressure of −15 cm H_2O indicates adequate respiratory muscle strength for weaning

580. High-frequency jet ventilation
1. can achieve adequate gas exchange when the tidal volume is less than the dead space volume
2. may be indicated for bronchopleural fistula
3. can be used during airway surgery
4. uses high driving pressures, which may cause barotrauma

581. The side effects of sedatives used in intensive care include
1. adrenal suppression with etomidate infusion
2. green urine with propofol
3. neuroleptic malignant syndrome with haloperidol
4. respiratory depression with midazolam

582. The complications of pulmonary artery catheterization include:
1. right bundle branch block
2. left bundle branch block
3. pulmonary artery rupture
4. bronchospasm

583. During mechanical ventilation the patient is able to take spontaneous breaths in which of the following modes?
1. assist/control (A/C)
2. intermittent mandatory ventilation (IMV)
3. synchronized intermittent mandatory ventilation (SIMV)
4. control mode ventilation (CMV)

584. In the multiple organ dysfunction syndrome (MODS)
1. the APACHE score may be an indicator of severity
2. the TISS score may be an indicator of severity
3. the most common cause is sepsis
4. failure of three systems carries a mortality of less than 50%

585. Which of the following statement(s) about parenteral nutrition is (are) true?
1. energy requirements may be increased two- to threefold in patients with large area burns
2. glucose, amino acids, fat, electrolytes, and vitamins may be mixed in a single bag for administration
3. delay in initiating nutrition may result in failure to wean from mechanical ventilation
4. fat emulsions may be administered via peripheral veins

586. Pulmonary thromboembolism
1. can be diagnosed from the clinical picture
2. may cause right heart failure
3. can be excluded if the PaO_2 is normal on room air
4. may cause an increase in $PaCO_2$ in mechanically ventilated patients

587. When gastric contents are aspirated into the lungs
1. increasing acidity (pH < 2.5) results in more severe lung damage
2. adult respiratory distress syndrome (ARDS) may develop
3. gastric acid may cause bronchospasm
4. keeping gastric pH neutral with antacids reduces nosocomial pneumonia

588. In disseminated intravascular coagulation
1. fibrinogen levels are normal or raised
2. there is an increase in clot formation
3. the platelet count is normal
4. there is bleeding due to coagulopathy

589. In a metabolic acidosis
1. there is a decrease in the bicarbonate level
2. the patient is hypoventilating
3. bicarbonate administration may cause a rise in $PaCO_2$
4. the pH may be greater than 7.44

590. Concerning pancreatitis
1. it may be a noninfectious cause of fever
2. it may occur following cardiopulmonary bypass

3. it can be complicated by ARDS
4. elevated serum amylase levels are more specific than lipase levels for making the diagnosis

591. In acetaminophen poisoning
1. treatment of overdose is effective up to three days later
2. N-acetylcysteine is effective in preventing the toxic effects
3. nephrotoxicity is the main toxic effect
4. acetaminophen levels should guide the necessity for treatment

592. In a patient in the ICU with renal failure, dialysis may be indicated by which of the following conditions?
1. fluid overload
2. hyperkalemia
3. uremia
4. hyperglycemia

593. In a patient who has suffered smoke inhalation
1. carbon monoxide poisoning causes cyanosis
2. high inspired oxygen concentrations should be avoided in carbon monoxide poisoning because of the risk of oxygen toxicity to the lungs
3. cyanide poisoning causes a reduction in mixed venous oxygen saturation
4. the PaO_2 may be normal in severe carbon monoxide toxicity

594. Pulmonary barotrauma
1. may be seen as pneumomediastinum
2. has an increased incidence in ventilated patients with low lung compliance
3. may cause subcutaneous emphysema
4. may cause pneumoperitoneum

595. With regard to colloid solutions
1. 5% albumin solution may cause a dilutional coagulopathy
2. hetastarch is primarily cleared by the liver
3. dextran "40" may cause renal failure
4. serum amylase levels may rise after hetastarch administration, indicating pancreatitis

596. Ranitidine, when given to ventilated ICU patients
1. directly blocks the acid pump in the gastric mucosal cells
2. may decrease the incidence of nosocomial pneumonia
3. must be given orally to reduce acid production by the stomach
4. is titrated to keep the gastric pH > 10

597. Prophylaxis against stress ulceration of the stomach in ventilated ICU patients may include
1. ranitidine
2. sucralfate
3. alkaline antacids
4. enteral feeding

598. If a patient is comatose from an unknown cause
1. thiamine should be given to prevent Wernicke's encephalopathy
2. IV glucose should be administered before the blood sugar result returns from the laboratory
3. naloxone should be administered
4. phenobarbital should be administered to prevent seizures

Intensive Care Unit

Answers and Discussion

The authors have made every effort to thoroughly verify the answers to the questions that appear on the preceding pages. As in any text, however, some inaccuracies and ambiguities may occur. If in doubt, please consult the indicated reference. When no page number(s) are cited, the reference is to a journal article or to a refresher course lecture that should be read in its entirety.

The Editors

566. **(D)** Because of increased fluid losses and inability to drink, patients in status asthmaticus may be severely dehydrated. Appropriate fluid administration is indicated. β_1 adrenergic agonists are cardioselective and therefore β_2 agonists, such as albuterol or terbutaline, should be used. High-dose intravenous or oral steroids should be used for the severe asthma attack. There is no role for inhaled steroids in this situation. Ipratroprium bromide is an anticholinergic agent that may be useful in combination with β_2 agonists. An increased dose of theophylline is required in smokers. (**Ref. 30,** pp. 331–340; **Ref. 20,** p. 1673)

567. **(C)** Alveolar edema occurs in ARDS as a result of extensive capillary leak. Hydrostatic pressure is increased in cardiogenic pulmonary edema. The lungs become stiff as the result of de-

creased compliance. Pancreatitis is commonly accompanied by poor oxygenation due to respiratory problems. In severe cases, this may progress to ARDS. The chest x-ray appearances may be similar, whatever the cause of the ARDS. PEEP may improve oxygenation by decreasing intrapulmonary shunting. (**Ref. 20,** pp. 1634–1647)

568. (D) When the intra-aortic balloon pump is being used, there is a reduction in preload during systole as a result of deflation of the balloon at the end of diastole. This results in lower pressure of assisted systole. Balloon inflation occurs during diastole and should be timed to start when the aortic valve closes. The increased diastolic pressure results in improved coronary perfusion. (**Ref. 23,** pp. 1127–1133)

569. (B) The key hemodynamic abnormality in septic shock is vasodilation. In the early stage this leads to a hyperdynamic state with tachycardia and a high cardiac output. The vasodilation also leads to a reduction in the effective circulating plasma volume, as shown by a reduced pulmonary capillary wedge pressure. Although oxygen delivery to the tissues may be normal or increased, systemic distribution of blood flow is abnormal and oxygen extraction is reduced, resulting in a raised SvO_2. (**Ref. 30,** pp. 177–180; **Ref. 20,** pp. 1173–1175)

570. (E) Oxygen delivery is the product of cardiac output and arterial oxygen content of the blood (CaO_2). Hypoxia causes a decrease in hemoglobin saturation, and this reduces the oxygen content of the blood. Hypovolemia decreases cardiac output, reducing oxygen delivery. An increase in oxygen consumption in the periphery will not cause any increase in the oxygen content of arterial blood or increase the cardiac output. Anemia reduces the oxygen-carrying capacity of the blood and reduces oxygen delivery. (**Ref. 30,** pp. 320–321; **Ref. 20,** pp. 3–8)

571. (C) The ulnar artery is not an end artery. It forms the palmar arches along with the radial artery. Sepsis is as common with arterial as with venous cannulae. An overly damped arterial tracing will reduce the pulse pressure with alterations in systolic and diastolic readings, but the mean arterial pressure will not be altered.

Cuff pressure readings are particularly prone to error in low-flow states. (**Ref. 30,** pp. 89–99; **Ref. 20,** pp. 318–321)

572. (D) Following trauma there is a latent interval of 12 to 72 hours before the development of the fat embolus syndrome. Lung injury is the most common manifestation, and fat globules may be identified in the sputum. Cerebral involvement that is a result of fat embolization as well as of hypoxia may lead to disorientation or coma. The characteristic rash occurs on the trunk and in the axillary folds, but the petechiae do not blanch with pressure. Early fixation of the fractures is the key in the management of fat embolus and should not be delayed, even if pulmonary involvement has developed. (**Ref. 20,** pp. 779–781, 1488–1489)

573. (C) To make the diagnosis of irreversible brain death, the cause of the coma must be known, and the presence of any reversible factors such as hypothermia must be excluded. Seizure activity is indicative of cerebral function and excludes the diagnosis. Decerebrate posturing requires a functioning brain stem and again excludes the diagnosis. Spinal reflexes may be retained in the presence of permanent and complete destruction of the brain stem and of the cerebral cortices. Their absence is not required to make the diagnosis. (**Ref. 30,** pp. 198–199, 659; **Ref. 20,** pp. 544, 1067)

574. (B) Amrinone is a phosphodiesterase inhibitor that decreases the intracellular breakdown of cAMP. It thus increases cAMP levels via a different mechanism than the beta adrenergic agonists. Its predominant action is vasodilation, but some positive inotropic effects may also be seen. Its adverse effects include thrombocytopenia, and this necessitates its withdrawal in the oral form. (**Ref. 30,** pp. 243–244; **Ref. 20,** p. 1587)

575. (B) The wide-complex tachycardias are most commonly ventricular in origin, but may be supraventricular with aberrant conduction. Amiodarone is a potent, second-line drug that is effective in ventricular and supraventricular tachycardias. Lidocaine is effective only in arrhythmias of ventricular origin. Procainamide is contraindicated in Torsades because it increases the QT interval and may aggravate the arrhythmia. The diagnosis of first-degree AV block requires a PR interval in excess of 0.2 sec. (**Ref. 30,** pp. 263–275; **Ref. 20,** pp. 1503–1520)

334 / 21: Intensive Care Unit

576. **(D)** Delirium or organic brain syndrome is commonly due to a physiological insult to the brain and may have a metabolic, anoxic, infective, or toxic basis. It is more common in the elderly. Delirium may appear as a wake/sleep cycle reversal and may also be exacerbated by sleep deprivation. The anticholinergic effects of amitriptyline may make the confusional state worse. Haloperidol is very useful in dealing with the delirious state, and the extrapyramidal side effects are unusual when it is administered intravenously. (Ref. 30, pp. 345–346; Ref. 20, pp. 1757–1767)

577. **(E)** Pseudomembranous colitis most commonly presents as watery diarrhea in patients on an antibiotic. It has been reported as a serious side effect, caused by almost any antibiotic, especially clindamycin. Vancomycin has not been reported to cause it and is effective in its treatment. The antibiotics eliminate the normal intestinal flora and *Clostridium difficile* proliferates, causing a diarrheal syndrome that develops into a severe colitis. (Ref. 30, pp. 64–67; Ref. 20, pp. 1351–1353)

578. **(C)** CAVH is very efficient at removing fluid. Extremely large volumes (as much as 15 liters/day) can be filtered, and care must be taken to replace this volume to avoid hypovolemia. CAVH requires anticoagulation and this may be a problem in ICU patients. Hemodialysis is the most efficient way of removing fluid and solutes; however, the rapid changes may cause hypotension and arrhythmias. Peritoneal dialysis is more gentle but may require prolonged or continuous use, and it also runs the risk of introducing infection. (Ref. 20, pp. 1920–1928)

579. **(A)** Malnutrition may contribute to respiratory muscle wasting and weakness, whereas an excessive carbohydrate load may increase the respiratory quotient and the minute volume required. Respiratory anxiety may increase oxygen demand and carbon dioxide production. This may be reduced by sedatives, but respiratory depression should be avoided. A maximum inspiratory pressure of -30 cm H_2O is considered the minimum to indicate adequate respiratory strength. Normal subjects can generate a pressure of -70 to -120 cm H_2O. (Ref. 30, pp. 399–409; Ref. 20, pp. 1626–1629)

580. (E) Gas exchange cannot be explained by conventional bulk flow in high-frequency ventilation because the tidal volume is less than dead-space volume. High-frequency ventilation may be very useful in ventilating patients with a bronchopleural fistula, because there is a more uniform distribution of ventilation. Ventilation may be achieved through a narrow cannula, allowing easy surgical access to the airway. The driving pressure of up to 50 psi means that barotrauma may easily occur if there is not a free route for expiration. (**Ref. 20,** pp. 150–151)

581. (E) Etomidate infusions have been shown to cause adrenal suppression with increased mortality. A metabolite of propofol turns the urine green, but this is of no consequence. The neuroleptic malignant syndrome may be caused by any butyrophenone or phenothiazine and is similar to the malignant hyperthermia syndrome. Although the benzodiazepines have a wide safety ratio compared with barbiturates, they may still cause respiratory depression. (**Ref. 30,** pp. 345–347; **Ref. 20,** pp. 966–968)

582. (B) A right bundle branch block may occur during insertion of a PA catheter. Although PA catheter insertion does not cause left bundle branch block by itself, if a left bundle branch block is already present, a complete heart block would result. In spite of this, the incidence of complete heart block is so low that it is not recommended to insert a temporary pacing wire in patients with left bundle branch block before the insertion of a PA catheter. Pulmonary artery rupture is the most serious complication of pulmonary artery catheterization. (**Ref. 20,** pp. 324–326)

583. (A) In CMV the inspiratory valve is closed between ventilator breaths so that no spontaneous breaths can be taken. In the assist/control mode, all spontaneous breaths are supplemented with a ventilator breath. In IMV and SIMV the inspiratory valve is open between mechanical breaths, allowing spontaneous breathing. (**Ref. 30,** pp. 371–373; **Ref. 20,** pp. 143–146)

584. (A) APACHE is an Acute Physiology and Chronic Health Evaluation tool, which can be used to assess the severity of MODS. The Therapeutic Intervention Scoring System (TISS) uses the amount of intervention or skilled care the patient receives as an indicator of the severity of illness. Sepsis is the most common precipitating illness for MODS. When the number of organ systems that have failed reaches three, the mortality is in the range of 80% to 100%. (**Ref. 30,** pp. 552, 613–618)

585. **(E)** Patients with large surface area burns may have extremely high calorie requirements. Energy needs may also be elevated in sepsis. The components of total parenteral nutrition may be mixed in a bag for ease of administration. Lack of nutritional support may lead to protein breakdown and muscle atrophy, and this has been implicated in weaning failure. Concentrated glucose solutions are hyperosmolar and should be given via a central vein if prolonged administration is anticipated. Lipid emulsions are relatively iso-osmolar with plasma and may be given peripherally. (**Ref. 30,** pp. 544–555; **Ref. 20,** pp. 1072–1079)

586. **(C)** The clinical presentation of pulmonary thromboembolism may be very unreliable and there are no consistent clinical findings. Hypoxia may be absent in 25% of the patients. Mechanical obstruction of the pulmonary artery and stimulation of humoral factors causing pulmonary vasoconstriction lead to raised pulmonary artery pressures, which in turn may lead to right heart failure. The dead space caused by the blockage of pulmonary arteries leads to a rise in $PaCO_2$ if the patient is unable to increase minute ventilation. (**Ref. 30,** pp. 80–81; **Ref. 20,** pp. 1476–1480)

587. **(A)** Animal research has suggested that the pH of the aspirated stomach contents is important in causing lung damage. When the pH of the stomach is kept neutral with antacids, however, gastric colonization may occur and may be a source for introducing bacteria into the pharynx. If these are aspirated past an endotracheal cuff, nosocomial pneumonia is more likely to result. Gastric acid is extremely irritating to the airway, and intense bronchospasm may result. ARDS is a common outcome after severe aspiration. (**Ref. 30,** p. 590; **Ref. 20,** pp. 1727–1731)

588. **(C)** The underlying problem in DIC is an increased propensity for clot formation. Consumption of the clotting factors by this process results in coagulopathic bleeding. Platelets and fibrin are consumed by the abnormal clotting, and the platelet count and fibrinogen levels are characteristically reduced. Part of the body's response to abnormal, disseminated coagulation is to break down the abnormal clot. This fibrinolysis results in a reduced fibrinogen level and increased fibrin degradation products (FDP). (**Ref. 20,** pp. 1827–1828)

589. (**B**) In any acidosis the pH will be below the normal range of 7.36 to 7.44. Compensation may return the pH toward but not beyond the normal. In a metabolic acidosis the normal response is hyperventilation to produce some respiratory compensation. Bicarbonate administration may increase the pH, but if the minute ventilation does not increase, then the metabolism of bicarbonate to H_2O and CO_2 will result in an increase in CO_2 production. (**Ref. 30,** pp. 416–421; **Ref. 20,** pp. 1955–1959)

590. (**A**) Many factors are implicated in the pathogenesis of pancreatitis, and it is not infrequently seen after cardiopulmonary bypass. Pulmonary problems are frequent and may progress to ARDS. Serum amylase may be elevated from other causes, and the serum lipase levels are more specific for pancreatitis. (**Ref. 20,** pp. 2028–2031)

591. (**C**) The main effect of acetaminophen poisoning is hepatotoxicity, which may be fatal. One of the metabolites of acetaminophen causes hepatocellular damage. The accumulation of this metabolite may be reduced by the administration of *N*-acetylcysteine. *N*-acetylcysteine is metabolized to glutathione, which has sulfhydryl groups that bind to the metabolite. *N*-acetylcysteine is effective only if given within 24 hours of the overdose. The need for treatment is guided by the acetaminophen levels, which are plotted on a nomogram. (**Ref. 20,** pp. 2136–2138)

592. (**A**) Fluid overload is the commonest indication for dialysis in the intensive care population, who may not respond to diuretic therapy. The management of hyperkalemia is facilitated by dialysis, though medical measures may still be required to protect the heart. Uremia causing CNS depression, platelet dysfunction and bleeding, or pericardial effusion may be treated with dialysis. The management of hyperglycemia is not altered by the presence of renal failure. (**Ref. 20,** pp. 1920–1921)

593. (**D**) Carboxyhemoglobin is bright red and the poisoned patient is characteristically cherry red in color. Although formation of carboxyhemoglobin reduces the oxygen-carrying capacity of blood, the Pao_2 may be normal. The mainstay of treatment is a high inspired oxygen concentration (100%) because this displaces carbon monoxide from hemoglobin and increases clearance. Cyanide paralyzes the cytochromes of the mitochondria by binding to ferric iron in the enzymes. This interrupts aerobic respiration, decreases oxygen consumption, and increases the SvO_2. (**Ref. 20,** pp. 2121–2122, 2125–2127)

594. **(E)** Pulmonary barotrauma occurs when an alveolus ruptures into the perivascular sheath and gas then dissects back along the vessels to the mediastinum. If the pressure of the gas increases in the mediastinum, the gas may decompress into the soft tissues causing subcutaneous emphysema, into the pleural cavity causing pneumothorax, or retroperitoneally into the abdomen. Patients with low pulmonary compliance are at increased risk, because of the increase in inflation pressures. (**Ref. 30,** pp. 390–391; **Ref. 20,** pp. 590–592)

595. **(B)** Albumin solution (plasma protein fraction, PPF) does not contain any coagulation factors; the albumin fraction has been separated and heat-treated so that it can be stored at room temperature for a prolonged period. Large volumes of albumen solution will, therefore, dilute the coagulation factors in the recipient's plasma. Hetastarch is cleaved by serum amylases and is then cleared mainly by the kidneys. The amylase levels may rise, but this is not indicative of pancreatitis. Dextran 40 may cause acute renal failure by inducing a hyperosmolar state in the glomerular blood. (**Ref. 30,** pp. 210–211)

596. **(D)** Ranitidine is a histamine (H_2) blocker that reduces gastric acid production. The dose should be adjusted to keep the pH > 4, since this level is thought to reduce the incidence of stress ulceration of the stomach. Oral or intravenous administration will be effective in reducing gastric acidity. The rise in pH may allow bacterial colonization of the normally sterile stomach and lead to transmission of organisms into the airway. (**Ref. 30,** pp. 59–60; **Ref. 20,** p. 602)

597. **(E)** Cimetidine is a histamine (H_2) blocker that reduces gastric acid production. The alkaline antacids can be used to alkalinize

the stomach, but require frequent measurement of gastric pH and 1 to 2 hourly dosing to keep the pH > 4. Sucralfate does not neutralize the gastric acid, but has a mucosal protectant effect. Enteral nutrition has been shown to reduce the incidence of gastric ulceration in the populations at risk. (**Ref. 30,** pp. 58–60; **Ref. 20,** p. 602)

598. (A) The management of the patient who is comatose from an unknown cause should include IV dextrose and this should be given immediately after the blood sugar sample is drawn. When glucose is administered to patients who are thiamine deficient (e.g., alcoholics), they may develop structural brain lesions in vulnerable areas of the brain, leading to Wernicke's encephalopathy. Naloxone is given to diagnose and treat opioid overdose. Anticonvulsants should be reserved for use in the patient having seizures. (**Ref. 20,** pp. 2051–2052, 2084–2086)

22
Medicolegal and Ethical Considerations

DIRECTIONS (Questions 599–602): Each of the questions or incomplete statements below is followed by five suggested answers or completions. Select the **one** that is best in each case.

599. The most frequent "damaging event" in malpractice litigation against anesthesiologists was
   A. cardiovascular collapse
   B. equipment failure
   C. convulsions
   D. respiratory problems
   E. wrong drug/dose administration

600. In the ASA study, the most common adverse outcome was death. The second most common outcome was
   A. nerve damage
   B. permanent brain damage
   C. airway trauma
   D. eye injury
   E. awareness/fright

601. Which of the following is NOT a duty of the health care provider?
- A. to practice at a professional level of care
- B. to make full disclosure
- C. to protect confidence
- D. to provide the very best possible care
- E. to offer continuing treatment

602. The elements of negligence do NOT include
- A. duty
- B. breach of duty
- C. damages
- D. assault and battery
- E. causation

DIRECTIONS (Questions 603–610): For each of the questions or incomplete answers below, **one** or **more** of the answers or completions are correct. Select
- A. if only 1, 2, and 3 are correct
- B. if only 1 and 3 are correct
- C. if only 2 and 4 are correct
- D. if only 4 is correct
- E. if all are correct

---

603. Good risk management is critical in reducing the malpractice problem. Its essential features include
1. identification of the problem
2. assessment of the problem
3. resolution of the problem
4. follow-up

604. Continuing care need not be provided if
1. the patient unilaterally terminates the relationship
2. the provider obtains a mutually acceptable substitute
3. the illness for which help was sought was successfully cured
4. the patient does not follow advice and does not pay reasonable bills

605. Which of the following is NOT an essential component of proper consent?
1. validity
2. freedom
3. informedness
4. in writing

606. Valid consent can be given by
1. spouse for an "incompetent" adult
2. legal parent for a minor child
3. adult sibling for a minor child
4. competent adult for himself/herself

607. In order to study an experimental drug, which of the following is required?
1. informed consent must be obtained
2. the patient must be a competent adult
3. the institutional review board (IRB) must grant approval
4. the patient's family must be informed

608. Who is responsible for ensuring the competence of the medical staff in a community hospital?
1. chief of the medical staff
2. chief executive officer of the hospital
3. chairmen of the respective departments
4. the hospital as a corporate entity

609. The decision to withdraw life support from a competent, conscious adult rests with
1. the family
2. the ethics committee of the institution
3. the attending physician
4. the patient

610. In a community hospital, there are one anesthesiologist and three nurse anesthetists. The latter are employees of the hospital. One of the nurses is clearly negligent in a case while the anesthesiologist is away on vacation. Where does the liability rest?
   1. the nurse
   2. the surgeon
   3. the anesthesiologist
   4. the hospital

Medicolegal and Ethical Considerations

Answers and Discussion

The authors have made every effort to thoroughly verify the answers to the questions that appear on the preceding pages. As in any text, however, some inaccuracies and ambiguities may occur. If in doubt, please consult the indicated reference. When no page number(s) are cited, the reference is to a journal article or to a refresher course lecture that should be read in its entirety.

The Editors

599. (D) In the ASA "Closed Claims Project" slightly more than 30% of all cases had problems with the respiratory system as the primary damaging event. Within this group 75% of all problems came from three preventable breaches of the standard of care. These were: inadequate ventilation (38%), unrecognized esophageal intubation (18%), and "difficult intubation" (17%). In the vast majority of the esophageal intubations (97%), it took 5 min or more before the error was recognized and any attempt at correction was made. In 48% of the esophageal intubations the record alleges that bilateral breath sounds were heard after intubation. Whether this represents an honest error or improper charting cannot be determined. In cases of difficult intubation only 38%

were found to include negligence. This compares with more than 80% in the esophageal intubation group. (**Ref. 6,** #211)

600. **(A)** Death was by far the most common adverse outcome, totaling 37% of all claims. The second most common adverse effect, with a total of 15%, was nerve injury. About 75% of these nerve injuries were contributed by only three specific nerve distributions. These were: the ulnar nerve (34%), the brachial plexus (23%), and the lumbosacral nerve roots (16%). It is interesting to note that it was impossible to determine the mechanism of the injury in many of these cases. Injury did occur even when all customary precautions were allegedly taken. A curious finding was that 69% of the claimants in ulnar nerve injury cases were male, and 60% of the patients filing for brachial plexus injury were female. Whether this indicates that for some unknown reason the male is more prone to ulnar nerve injury could be the basis of some intriguing speculation and, perhaps, some rewarding research. (**Ref. 6,** #211)

601. **(D)** It is the duty of the health care provider to practice at least at the level of care of similar practitioners working under identical or similar circumstances. Practitioners are not expected to work at the highest possible level, although the practitioners may set higher standards than the national norm. If they do, they are bound to the self-set high standards. The duty of full disclosure has been repeatedly stated by a variety of courts. Basically, the "patient is entitled to know." Since the patient–provider relationship is a fiduciary one, keeping confidential all information concerning the patient is an absolute rule, unless there are statutory exemptions, such as bullet wounds, child abuse, certain infectious diseases, and so on. Continuing treatment must be provided unless the health care provider has a legitimate excuse to formally terminate the relationship. (See #609.) (**Ref. 12,** pp. 12–13, 27)

602. **(D)** The four elements that the patient must prove by a preponderance of evidence are duty, breach of duty, damages, and proximate causation. This means that there has to be a patient–provider professional relationship, that the standards of care expected from this practitioner have been violated, that there were damages, and, finally, that the damages were the direct result of the breach of the standard of care. Assault and battery in medical malpractice

comes under the heading of intentional tort and not under negligence, which is an unintentional tort. Assault and battery means, in this general context, that the provider did something to the patient without the patient's knowledge and permission. (**Ref. 35,** pp. 7, 19)

603. (**E**) The four elements listed in #602 are the essential components of good risk management. As soon as a problem (or potential problem) is identified—as soon as it is realized either that something bad has happened or that a given situation or practice represents a potential hazard to the patient—the risk manager must be notified. The risk manager and the physicians and nurses involved in the incident will assess and evaluate the problem. They determine how serious the injury or threat of injury may be and also how urgently the resolution of the problem must be accomplished. The third step is the resolution, namely, the establishment of proper safeguards to reasonably assure the institution that the problem will not again occur. The last steps are the retrospective assessment of the success of the process and making certain that the remedial steps continue to be enforced. Risk management includes such wide-ranging areas as proper credentialing and disciplinary procedures, equipment maintenance, record keeping and record review, efficient and meaningful death and complication conferences, and responsiveness to adverse events. (**Ref. 6,** #422)

604. (**A**) The duties of the health care providers include the provision of continuing care. The patient may terminate this relationship unilaterally and for no reason at all, but the health care provider may not. The circumstances under which the relationship may be terminated are clearly defined. Obviously, if the patient terminates the relationship, no further duty rests on the physician. Other ways of terminating the professional relationship are finding a mutually acceptable substitute who is willing to accept the patient, completion of the treatment that brought the patient to the provider, formal notice of termination by the provider by some provable route (certified mail, return receipt requested), and provision of adequate time for the patient to find a substitute. Nonpayment of fees or noncompliance with advice and instruction are not sufficient excuse to break the relationship without going through the formal termination process. (**Ref. 12,** pp. 12–13)

605. (A) The consent must be valid (i.e., it must be given by a person who is legally authorized to do so). It must be freely given (i.e., it must be obtained without any coercion and by a person for whom the refusal to consent does not constitute any threat of reprisal—prisoners, for example). It must be informed (i.e., the person giving the consent must understand, as well as possible under the circumstances, what is consented to and the consequences of consenting or withholding consent). It is frequently not possible to get a truly and fully informed consent from a lay person, but reasonable attempts must be made to advise the patient of the possible major complications, particularly if these are life-threatening or if they would seriously affect the patient's quality of life. Consent need not be in writing. Verbal agreement is perfectly legal, although it may be more difficult to prove. (**Ref. 21,** pp. 225 et seq.)

606. (C) The only persons who can give valid consent are competent adults of legal age in the jurisdiction where the treatment takes place, legal parents of a minor child, and court-appointed guardians for an adult declared incompetent. Emancipated minors may also give valid consent for themselves, and there may be statutory regulations governing the right of nonemancipated minors to give valid consent for therapy under carefully defined circumstances (VD, pregnancy). Except in Michigan, where there is statutory authority for a legal spouse to consent on behalf of an "incompetent" spouse, the family has no standing in such matters. It may be good practice to advise the family about the contemplated procedure, but the parents of legal adults and the adult siblings of minor children have no legal right to grant or to withhold consent. (**Ref. 12,** pp. 82–83)

607. (B) The only difference between consent for an experimental procedure and any traditional procedure is that approval for the experimental procedure must come from the Institutional Review Board (IRB). This board evolved from federal regulations, following scandalous human experiments having been performed without adequate consent from the patients who unknowingly served as experimental subjects. The IRB must review the proposed research protocol and rule on the appropriateness of the proposal, including the type of information that must be provided to the prospective subjects of the study. (**Ref. 21,** p. 258)

608. (D) Traditionally, the hospital had only to provide a safe and suitable environment for the independently practicing physicians to take care of their patients. The liability for negligence rested exclusively on the physician or vicariously on the hospital if the tort-feasor was an employee. All this was changed drastically by the celebrated Darling decision in Illinois in 1965 and by a substantial number of similar opinions in other jurisdictions since that time. Currently the governing board of the hospital is responsible for the quality of care provided by the physician staff members of the hospital, even though there is no employer–employee relationship between the institution and the physician. (**Ref. 35,** pp. 203–204)

609. (D) This is another situation in which the family, the ethics committee, and the physicians have no legal standing. The patient is the sole arbiter of his or her fate. The decision to terminate life support can and must be made by the conscious, competent patient alone. If the patient is not competent to make the decision, the physicians must do so. In this situation, many institutions require that the ethics committee be asked for advice. (**Ref. 12,** pp. 82–83)

610. (D) The nurse is likely to be included in the complaint, but technically the nurse is an employee of the hospital and, hence, the hospital is liable vicariously for the negligence of the employee. Since anesthesia is the practice of medicine, it can be practiced only by a nonphysician (nurse, dentist, etc.) under the delegatory clause of the code and under the supervision of a licensed physician. When the surgeon is the only physician present, he or she may well be held liable for failure to adequately supervise. The anesthesiologist's liability is negligible in this situation, unless he or she knew or should have known that the nurse was incompetent. (**Ref. 7,** p. 119; **Ref. 35,** pp. 665–675)

References

1. Abram ES: *The Pain Clinic Manual.* Philadelphia, JB Lippincott, 1991.
2. Altman DG: "Statistics and ethics in medical research," *British Medical Journal,* 281:1336–1338, 1980.
3. American Society of Anesthesiology Refresher Course Manual, 1989.
4. American Society of Anesthesiology Refresher Course Manual, 1990.
5. American Society of Anesthesiology Refresher Course Manual, 1991.
6. American Society of Anesthesiology Refresher Course Manual, 1993.
7. Barash PG, Cullen BF, Stoelting RK: *Clinical Anesthesia,* 2nd ed. Philadelphia, JB Lippincott, 1992.
8. Blitt C (ed): *Invasive Blood Pressure Monitoring,* 2nd ed. New York, Churchill Livingstone, 1990.
9. Bonica JJ: *The Management of Pain,* 2nd ed. Philadelphia, Lea & Febiger, 1990.
10. Cote CJ: *A Practice of Anesthesia for Infants and Children,* 2nd ed. Philadelphia, WB Saunders, 1993.
11. Cousins MJ, Bridenbaugh PO: *Neural Blockade in Clinical Anesthesia and Management of Pain,* 2nd ed. Philadelphia, JB Lippincott, 1988.

12. Dornette WHL (ed): *Legal Issues in Anesthesia Practice.* Philadelphia, FA Davis Company, 1991.
13. Eichhorn JH, Ehrenwert J: *Anesthesia Equipment: Principles and Applications.* Chicago, Mosby-Yearbook, 1993.
14. Frost AME: *Clinical Anesthesia in Neurosurgery,* 2nd ed. Oxford, Butterworth-Heinemann, 1991.
15. Goodman, Gilman: *The Pharmacological Basis of Therapeutics,* 8th ed. Goodman AG et al (eds). New York, Pergamon Press, 1990.
16. Grabb WC, Smith JW (eds): *Plastic Surgery,* 4th ed. Boston, Little Brown, 1991.
17. Gravlee JE et al (eds): *Cardiopulmonary Bypass: Principles and Practice.* Baltimore, Williams and Wilkins, 1993.
18. *Gray's Anatomy,* 37th ed. New York, Churchill Livingstone, 1989.
19. Gregory GA: *Pediatric Anesthesia,* 2nd ed. New York, Churchill Livingstone, 1989.
20. Hall JB, Schmidt GA, Wood LDH: *Principles of Critical Care.* New York, McGraw-Hill, 1992.
21. Holder AR: *Medical Malpractice Law,* 2nd ed. New York, John Wiley and Sons, 1978.
22. *Harrison's Principles of Internal Medicine,* 13th ed. Wilson et al (eds). New York, McGraw-Hill, 1994.
23. Kaplan JA (ed): *Cardiac Anesthesia,* 3rd ed. Philadelphia, WB Saunders Company, 1993.
24. Kaplan JA (ed): *Thoracic Anesthesia,* 2nd ed. New York, Churchill Livingstone, 1991.
25. Kaplan JA (ed): *Vascular Anesthesia.* New York, Churchill Livingstone, 1991.
26. Katz J, Benumoff JL, Kadis LB (eds): *Anesthesia and Uncommon Diseases,* 3rd ed. Philadelphia, WB Saunders, 1990.
27. Lake C: *Clinical Monitoring.* Philadelphia, WB Saunders, 1990.
28. Lake C: *Pediatric Cardiac Anesthesia.* Norwalk, Appleton & Lange, 1988.
29. McGoldrick K: *Anesthesia for Ophthalmic and Otorlaryngologic Surgery.* Philadelphia, WB Saunders, 1992.
30. Marino PL: *The ICU Book.* Philadelphia, Lea and Febiger, 1991.
31. Maurer K, Lowitzsch K, Stöhr M: *Evoked Potentials,* Toronto, BC Decker, 1989.
32. Miller RD (ed): *Anesthesia,* 3rd ed. New York, Churchill Livingstone, 1990.

33. Mushin WW, Jones PL (eds): *Physics for the Anaesthetist*, 4th ed. Boston, Blackwell Scientific Publications, 1987.
34. Norris MC (ed): *Obstetric Anesthesia*. Philadelphia, JB Lippincott Company, 1993.
35. Peters JD et al: *Anesthesiology and the Law*. Ann Arbor, Health Administration Press, 1983.
36. Rogers MC, Tinker JH, Covino BG, Longnecker DE: *Principles and Practice of Anesthesiology*. Chicago, Mosby-Yearbook, 1993.
37. Roizen M (ed): *Anesthesia for Vascular Surgery*. New York, Churchill Livingstone, 1990.
38. Schneider SM, Levenson G (eds): *Anesthesia for Obstetrics*, 3rd ed. Baltimore, Williams & Wilkins, 1993.
39. Smith RM: *Anesthesia for Infants and Children*, 5th ed. St. Louis, CV Mosby, 1990.
40. Stoelting RK, Dierdorf SF, McCammon RL: *Anesthesia and Coexisting Disease*, 2nd ed. New York, Churchill Livingstone, 1988.
41. Stoelting RK: *Pharmacology and Physiology in Anesthesia Practice*, 2nd ed. Philadelphia, JB Lippincott, 1991.
42. Thomas SJ (ed): *Manual of Cardiac Anesthesia*, 2nd ed. New York, Churchill Livingstone, 1993.
43. Vander AJ, Sherman JH, Luciano DS: *Human Physiology*, 6th ed. New York, McGraw-Hill, 1994.
44. Voet D, Voet JG: *Biochemistry*. New York, John Wiley and Sons, 1990.
45. Warfield AC: *Principles and Practices of Pain*. New York, McGraw-Hill, 1993.
46. Wedel DJ: *Orthopedic Anesthesia*. New York, Churchill Livingstone, 1993.
47. Wetchler BV: *Anesthesia for Ambulatory Surgery*, 2nd ed. Philadelphia, JB Lippincott, 1991.

Glossary of Abbreviations

AA	Alcoholics Anonymous
ABG	Arterial blood gases
A/C	Assist/control
AC	Alternating current
ACE	Acetylcholinesterase
ACh	Acetylcholine
ACOG	American College of Obstetrics and Gynecology
ACT	Active coagulation time
ADH	Antidiuretic hormone
AIDS	Acquired immunodeficiency syndrome
ALA	Aminolevulinic acid
ALT	Alanine aminotransferase
AP	Anteroposterior
APACHE	Acute Physiology and Chronic Health Evaluation
aPTT	Activated prothrombin time
ARDS	Adult Respiratory Distress Syndrome
ARF	Acute renal failure
ASA	American Society of Anesthesiology
ASD	Atrial septal defect
AST	Aspartate aminotransferase
ATP	Adenosine triphosphate
AV	Atrioventricular

AVSD	Atrioventricular septal defect
BBB	Blood–brain barrier
BMR	Basal metabolic rate
BP	Blood pressure
BSO	Bilateral salpingo-oophorectomy
BV	Blood volume
C	Celsius
CABG	Coronary artery bypass graft
CAD	Coronary artery disease
CaM	Calmodulin
cAMP	Cyclic adenosine monophosphate
CAVH	Continuous arteriovenous hemofiltration
CBF	Cerebral blood flow
CBV	Cerebral blood volume
CC	Closing capacity
CCBF	Critical cerebral blood flow
cGMP	Cyclic guanine monophosphate
CHF	Congestive heart failure
CMR	Cerebral metabolic rate
$CMRO_2$	Cerebral metabolic rate for oxygen
CMV	Control mode ventilation
CMV	Cytomegalovirus
CNS	Central nervous system
CO	Cardiac output
CO	Carbon monoxide
CoA	Coenzyme A
COMT	Catechol-O-methyl transferase
COPD	Chronic obstructive pulmonary disease
CPAP	Continuous positive airway pressure
CPB	Cardiopulmonary bypass
CPP	Cerebral perfusion pressure
CR	Creatinine
CRF	Chronic renal failure
CSF	Cerebrospinal fluid
CT	Computer tomography
CVP	Central venous pressure
D&C	Dilatation and curettage
D&E	Dilatation and evacuation
DC	Direct current
DCR	Dacro-cysto-rhinostomy
DIC	Disseminated intravascular coagulation

DNA	Deoxyribonucleic acid
DO_2	Oxygen delivery
DOPA	3,4 Dihydroxyphenylalanine
DPG	Diphosphoglycerate
DVT	Deep venous thrombosis
EACA	Epsilon amino caproic acid
ECG	Electrocardiogram(ph)
EEG	Electroencephalogram
EMG	Electromyography
ENT	Ear, nose, and throat
ESI	Epidural steroid injection
ESWL	Extracorporeal shock wave lithotripsy
ET	Endotracheal
F	Fahrenheit
FDA	Food and Drug Administration
FDP	Fibrin degradation products
FES	Fat embolism syndrome
FEV	Forced expiratory volume
FFP	Fresh-frozen plasma
FRC	Functional residual capacity
FVC	Forced vital capacity
GA	Gestational age
GABA	Gamma amino butyric acid
GFR	Glomerular filtration rate
GHRH	Growth hormone releasing hormone
GI	Gastrointestinal
GIP	Gastric inhibitory peptide
GIP	Glucose-dependent insulinotropic peptide
GMP	Guanine monophosphate
GTP	Guanine triphosphate
Hb	Hemoglobin
HbS	Hemoglobin S
Hct	Hematocrit
HDL	High-density lipoprotein
HELLP	Hemolysis, elevated liver enzymes, low platelet count
HLA	Histocompatibility lymphocytic antigen
HLHS	Hypoplastic left heart syndrome
HPV	Hypoxic pulmonary vasoconstriction
HR	Heart rate
Hz	Hertz
I-E ratio	Inspiratory-expiratory ratio

IABP	Intraaortic ballooon pump
ICP	Intracranial pressure
ICU	Intensive care unit
IDM	Infant of diabetic mother
IgE	Immunoglobulin E
IgG	Immunoglobulin G
IgM	Immunoglobulin M
IMV	Intermittent mandatory ventilation
IOP	Intraocular pressure
IP	Interphalangeal
IRB	Institutional review board
IRV	Inspiratory reserve volume
IUGR	Intrauterine growth retarded
IV	Intravenous
LDL	Low-density lipoprotein
LGA	Large for gestational age
LMA	Laryngeal mask airway
LTB	Laryngotracheo bronchitis (croup)
LVEDP	Left ventricular end-diastolic pressure
LV	Left ventricle
ms	Millisecond
mA	Milliampere
MAC	Minimum anesthetic concentration
MAO	Monoamine oxidase
MAP	Mean arterial pressure
MH	Malignant hyperthermia
MI	Myocardial infarction
MODS	Multiple organ dysfunction syndrome
MPS	Myofascial pain syndrome
MR	Mitral regurgitation
MRI	Magnetic resonance imaging
MVV	Maximum voluntary ventilation
NADH	Reduced form of nicotinamide adenine dinucleotide
NICU	Neonatal intensive care unit
NMDA	N-methyl-d-spartase
NPH	Neutral protamine Hagedorn (insulin)
NPO	Nil per os (nothing by mouth)
NSAID	Nonsteroidal antiinflammatory drug
NYHA	New York Heart Association
OA	Osteoarthritis
P	Pressure

Glossary of Abbreviations / 357

PACU	Postanesthesia care unit
PAD	Pulmonary artery diastolic pressure
PCA	Post-conceptual age
PA	Pulmonary artery
$PaCO_2$	Arterial carbon dioxide tension
PaO_2	Arterial oxygen tension
PCP	Phencyclidine hydrochloride
PDA	Patent ductus arteriosus
PDPH	Post dural puncture headache
PE	Pulmonary embolus (embolization)
PEEP	Positive endexpiratory pressure
PET	Positive emission tomography
PFT	Pulmonary function test
PGR	Psychogalvanic reflex
PI	Proximal interphalangeal
PKP	Penetrating keratoplasty
PPF	Plasma protein fraction
PP	Pump prime volume
psi	Pounds per square inch
PSIG	Pounds per square inch gauge pressure
PT	Prothrombin time
PTT	Partial prothrombin time
PVC	Premature ventricular contraction
PVR	Pulmonary vascular resistance
RA	Rheumatoid arthritis
RBC	Red blood cell
RINDS	Reversible ischemic neurologic deficits
RNA	Ribonucleic acid
ROP	Retinopathy of prematurity
RSD	Reflex sympathetic dystrophy
RV	Right ventricle
RVEDP	Right ventricular end-diastolic presssure
SA	Sinoauricular
SaO_2	Arterial oxygen saturation
SEP	Somatosensory evoked potential
SGA	Small for gestational age
SIMV	Synchronized intermittent mandatory ventilation
SMP	Sympathetically maintained pain
SvO_2	Mixed venous oxygen saturation
SVR	Systemic vascular resistance
SVT	Superventricular tachycardia

TAH	Total abdominal hysterectomy
TEF	Tracheoesophageal fistula
TENS	Transcutaneous electrical nerve stimulation
TGA	Transposition of great arteries
TH	Thyrotropic hormone
THA	Total hip arthroplasty
TIA	Transient ischemic attack
TISS	Therapeutic intervention scoring system
TMJ	Temporomandibular joint
TOF	Tetralogy of Fallot
TRAM	Transverse rectus abdominis musculocutaneous flap
TURP	Transurethral prostatectomy
U.K.	United Kingdom
V	Volume
VAE	Venous air embolism
VC	Vital capacity
VLDL	Very low-density lipoprotein
V/Q	Ventilation perfusion ratio
VSD	Ventricular septal defect
VT	Ventricular tachycardia
VVO	Ventricle pace, ventricle sense, O inhibition pacemaker